Sidney Cohen

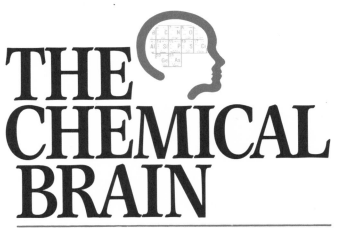

THE CHEMICAL BRAIN

The Neurochemistry

Of Addictive Disorders

Forewords by Robert L. DuPont, M.D.
and David E. Smith, M.D.

CareInstitute
Irvine, California

Library of Congress Cataloging-in-Publication Data
Cohen, Sidney, 1910-1987
    The chemical brain.

    Bibliography: p.
    1. Substance abuse—Pathophysiology.   2. Substance abuse—Chemotherapy.
3. Substance abuse—Genetic aspects.   4. Neurophysiology.   I. Title. [DNLM:
1. Brain—drug effects.   2. Brain Chemistry.   3. Psychotropic Drugs—
pharmacokinetics.   4. Substance Abuse.   WL 300 C678]
RC564.C625   1988   616.86'071   88-6036
ISBN 0-917877-01-0

Cover design by Lillian Svec

Requests for additional copies should be addressed to
CompCare Publishers
2415 Annapolis Lane
Minneapolis, MN 55441
Call toll free 800/328-3330
(Minnesota residents 612/559-4800)

2	3	4	5	6
89	90	91	92	93

Contents

Foreword by David E. Smith, M.D.
   "In Memoriam: Sidney Cohen, M.D"
Foreword by Robert L. DuPont, M.D.
   "The Legacy of Sidney Cohen"

Preface

Tables & Figures

In Memoriam:
Sidney Cohen, M.D.

The death of Sidney Cohen, M.D., has created a deep void in the drug abuse field. Sidney Cohen was the elder statesman and the most rational voice in the very irrational world of drugs in the United States.

In the 1960s, when the viewpoints of many professionals became too liberal regarding the use of drugs, Sidney Cohen's guidance helped those professionals in a fledgling field to become more objective, particularly in relation to the "tune in, turn on, drop out" philosophy. In the 1980s, when the voices of the right wing promoted character assassination and the inaccessibility of drug information as well as an antitreatment, proincarceration philosophy, Sidney Cohen spoke out against this extreme conservatism, as he had done before against earlier liberal excesses.

On a personal level, Sidney Cohen was very influential in my life and professional career. His teaching syllabus in psychopharmacology in the early 1960s was one of my key references in this area. He provided a rational basis for the toxicity of a variety of drugs—including marijuana, LSD, and cocaine—that was used as a guideline at the Haight-Ashbury Free Medical Clinic. His book on LSD, *The Beyond Within*, became one of the most important references in the mid-1960s for gaining an understanding of the complicated world of psychedelic drugs.

Sidney Cohen taught us that marijuana was a lot more dangerous than we originally thought, particularly with the use of more potent preparations by young people. He referred conceptual battles, such as who developed the term "amotivational syndrome," to their appropriate clinical, rather than political, applications. Sidney Cohen not only served government in the drug abuse field, but he advised government not to lose control to extremists who made drug abuse a political issue, even though his warning might not have been popular at the time.

In *The Chemical Brain*, Sidney Cohen chronicles recent advances in science relative to brain chemistry. These advances have been nothing less than phenomenal. We have taken quantum leaps in our understanding of drugs and the people who abuse or are addicted to drugs. For instance, our understanding of brain chemistry has recently provided us with knowledge about opiate, benzodiazepine, and other receptor sites which allow us incredible insight into the development of addiction and the pharmacologic requirements for detoxification from those drugs. In addition, the study of brain chemistry has taught us much relative to the development of pharmacologic treatment rationales for the postdetox recovery process. Equally important has been the insight that we have gained about the neurochemistry of people who are at risk for addiction. We have learned that any reason to study drugs and drug abuse necessarily takes into account not only the specific psychopharmacology of the drug but also host factors, including the study of the genetic effects of addiction.

The American Medical Association recently stated that all chemical dependencies are diseases, not just alcoholism. Within the field of chemical dependency treatment, it has long been felt that there was a commonality among all of the addictions and that the link between addicts and alcoholics was stronger than any pharmacologically specific differences. In other words, what is important is a refocusing on the broader issues that underlie all addictive behavior, while focusing on the specific psychopharmacology of a drug for specific treatment modalities, e.g., the use of amino acids for cocaine withdrawal and recovery or the use of naltrexone and opiate agonists used in opiate recovery. Clearly, a comprehensive or holistic view of chemical dependency rests squarely upon the study of brain chemistry.

This book is an excellent window on the subject of neurochemistry, which is clearly where the most remarkable and fundamental progress is being made relative to the understanding and treatment of addictive disease. Sidney Cohen was a pioneer in the scholarly inquiry into the causes and treatment of addictive disease, and *The Chemical Brain* is an excellent example of his dedication and important contributions to the relatively young field of addictionology.

Sidney Cohen took the long view and tempered scientific objectivity with humanism. He was a great source of knowledge, inspiration and guidance, and he will be profoundly missed. However, his spirit lives on and will continue to motivate those of us in the drug abuse field to try to find rational solutions to this country's alcohol and other drug abuse problems.

David E. Smith, M.D.
Founder and Medical Director
Haight-Ashbury Free Medical Clinics
San Francisco, California

The Legacy of Sidney Cohen

When I first met Sidney Cohen, M.D., in 1970, I was the Director of the Narcotics Treatment Administration (NTA), Washington, D.C.'s heroin addiction treatment program. Methadone was a central part of our treatment approach. This policy was terribly controversial at the time—the common criticism being that we were "just replacing one addiction with another." Most of the medical and virtually all of the federal health bureaucracy was then "antimethadone."

One day I was asked to speak at the National Naval Medical Center in Bethesda about NTA's innovative program. I arrived at the meeting in time to hear the speaker who preceded me on the program, Sidney Cohen, speak on the uses and abuses of methadone in the treatment of heroin addiction. He was then the head of the Division of Narcotics Addiction and Drug Abuse (DNADA), in the National Institute for Mental Health (NIMH).

Not knowing Dr. Cohen, I came prepared to listen to the usual bureaucratic foolishness. I sat in the back of the room prepared to take the podium next, to defend myself and the NTA program. I listened, at first with half an ear, but after Dr. Cohen's opening remarks, I sat up in my seat, fully alert. I had listened to many talks about the treatment of heroin addiction over the previous three years but I had never heard anything like I heard that day. With good humor, wisdom, and insight, Dr. Cohen simply presented the problems and the solutions. All the conflict-driven members of the audience—those who were "promethadone" as well as those who were "antimethadone" (in those days there weren't many who weren't one or the other!)—listened and learned, calmly and with pleasure. When it came my turn to speak I began by saying that I had never before heard such a lucid description of the current state of knowledge about heroin addiction treatment. I left the platform and introduced myself to Dr. Cohen. He said something like "It's nice to meet you. Thank you for your kind words but, really, anyone here could have done what I did. I just went over the facts as they are generally known these days."

That was my first meeting with Sidney Cohen. Over the years our paths crossed many, many times. When I was Director of the National Institute on Drug Abuse (NIDA), I had some good moments and some bad ones. The best of the good ones were when Sidney Cohen came to Washington from his home in California. He was always welcome in my office. He would come in and ask me how I was doing—usually laughing good-naturedly at my most recent windmill bashing. I would ask him to sort out a problem for me—it was always something that I had puzzled over and that our entire research staff had puzzled over. He was unfailingly a good, kind, and marvelously wise teacher.

At one point in the mid-1970s we at NIDA were concerned but ill-informed about the problem of inhalant abuse. Once again a lot of obvious foolishness was then being circulated by drug abuse professionals, as it had been a few years earlier about methadone treatment of heroin addicts. Sidney Cohen accepted my invitation to write a report on inhalant abuse. He completed in a few weeks a short but complete report summarizing the current state of knowledge, not only ending most of the controversy but also pointing us in the direction of improved programs and policies.

When I left NIDA to join the American Council for Drug Education (ACDE), there was an urgent need for useful and reliable information about the health hazards of marijuana and cocaine. Sidney Cohen wrote ACDE monographs on the effects of marijuana smoking on the lungs and on the problems caused by cocaine. The scientists working in these controversial areas were not only at each other's throats, but they were incensed by the misstatements in the popular and even much of the professional press on the subjects. In each case Sidney Cohen stepped in, sorted it out, wrote a cogent report, and moved on. He did the same on the subject of the uses and abuses of benzodiazepines—medicines like Valium and Xanax.

Dr. Cohen not only wrote reports and books, he traveled the globe speaking and sharing his knowledge about drugs. I marveled at his flexibility as he got off transcontinental flights and took up the task at hand without missing a beat.

Once I commented to him about his role in the drug abuse field: I saw him as the trusted wise man in a field filled with lots of smoke but little light. No one else, literally, could think and write the way Sidney Cohen did. No one else commanded such broad respect from the most prodrug to the most antidrug zealots. When Sidney Cohen dealt with a topic, what he said was simply the way it was. He modestly rejected my praise. He felt that his contributions were similar to those made by many others. He never, at least not to my knowledge, appreciated his own unique value to all of us struggling not only to understand but to help solve drug abuse problems. By contrast, I never met anyone, from any political or ideological camp, who did not like and admire Sidney Cohen.

I have probably made him seem like a sort of Jimmy Stewart intellectual. He was not "laid back" or casual about himself or his ideas. He was warm and enormously generous but he was always the professional. He had what seemed to me to be great, but not uncritical, respect for everyone who cared about the drug problem. He was a man without enemies in a field filled with hostility. He surely did not agree with me on many topics. He was quite willing—more honestly I could say he was eager—to tell me where and why we differed. For example, I have consistently been an enthusiastic supporter of urine testing as part of a comprehensive drug abuse prevention program in the workplace and in schools. Noting that there were many, many ways to dupe the urine screening procedures as they are commonly performed, especially in the workplace, Dr. Cohen said, "I am not sure urine testing will identify drug use, but I am certain that it will detect stupidity."

Sidney Cohen, unlike many of us who came after him, did not start his career with the 1960s drug epidemic. He graduated with a degree in pharmacy from Columbia University in 1930 even before he received his bachelor's degree from City College in New York in 1932. He took his medical training at Bonn University in Germany, getting an M.D. degree in 1938, and then completed his postgraduate medical training back in the United States. I can only guess at what it must have been like for him to study medicine in Nazi Germany in the 1930s!

Dr. Cohen's first publications were about medical problems, but from the onset two characteristics were evident in his writing: the breadth of his interests and his commitment to his initial field of pharmacology. The first sign from his awe-inspiring resume of his later involvement with chemical dependence came in 1958 with the thirteenth professional publication in his career, "Subjective Reports of LSD—25 Experiences in a Context of Psychological Test Performance." This paper was published in the *American Journal of Psychiatry*. His next paper, also published in 1958, was one of the early studies of the class of drugs which was to change the lives of psychotic psychiatric patients throughout the world as he wrote about the uses of a new phenothiazine medication. This combination of abused and therapeutic drugs was, for Dr. Cohen, an expression of his abiding interest in pharmacology. Sidney Cohen sought to understand how drugs affected people, with drug abusers and in medical patients.

As the decade of the 1960s progressed he began to speak on college campuses all over the country in a debate format with Timothy Leary, the "Harvard professor" who was the Pied Piper of the drug epidemic. Even in those early years, before most professionals caught even a glimmer of what was to come, Sidney Cohen was sounding the warning about the dangers of using chemicals to have fun or to "expand consciousness."

I understand that Timothy Leary retains a great respect for Sidney Cohen. From the point that Dr. Cohen entered into this adversarial relationship with Leary, his career became far more complex than can be related in this foreword. In summary, from that time until the end of his life Sidney Cohen was at the center of every important development in the drug abuse field. He was a teacher, a researcher, a clinician, and a bureaucrat by turns, bringing great distinction to each role.

During the last year of his life he became excited and preoccupied with his work on *The Chemical Brain*. During my last meeting with him, shortly before his tragic and completely unexpected death, he talked about his project with an enthusiasm I had never heard from him on any of his many previous intellectual missions. He would, he told me, summarize the current state of knowledge about the way the brain worked, using new scientific knowledge to explain drug abuse in new and useful ways.

Throughout the last two decades of the drug abuse epidemic in the United States much of the discussion of the issue has been in terms of policies and programs and politics and religion. What most of the public has not noticed is that the most important development over this period is not related to any of these approaches. The most important and enduring part of the global response to the drug problem has been intellectual, as researchers around the world have sought to understand why people use drugs and what drugs do in the brain.

In 1973, when I was the new head of NIDA and Sidney Cohen was my number one guru, a historic development took place: NIDA-funded researchers found that there was a specific receptor in the brain for morphine. Shortly thereafter it was discovered that there were natural brain chemicals that fit these receptors. That finding opened the door to new understanding of not only how abused drugs worked, but how the brain worked. In fact, many people, certainly including me, believed that this search for understanding the brain, most of which grew directly out of research into how abused drugs worked, was the most important frontier of modern biology. Several of our colleagues who made original contributions to this new knowledge are likely to win Nobel Prizes within the next few years for their work.

As the research was published, Sidney Cohen became more and more excited by it. It was, he felt, as if all his life's work could, at long last, be fit together like the pieces from a puzzle. Many pieces he knew remained to be discovered. But many of the most important pieces were found in recent years. Sidney Cohen took up the task of writing *The Chemical Brain* with the zest of a man half his age. He wrote rapidly with complete command of the material. Here, truly, was an opportunity for him to use the full range of the knowledge he had built up over five decades of study.

He left us, in this book, a legacy. It is his testament and his last gift to all of us. In it is wisdom and enlightenment for people who are interested in either drug abuse or in the ways the brain works. Sidney Cohen in this book writes for the mental health professional, the chemical dependence expert, and the interested reader of modern science.

He is here at the peak of his skills as he explains the most complicated current science with a clarity and simplicity that make it available and authentic to both the novice and the expert. Dr. Cohen had a unique ability to simplify complex ideas in ways that did not diminish or distort their full importance. The most arcane scientific papers became clear when Sidney Cohen wrote about them.

Let me end, as I began, on a personal note. I knew and loved Sidney Cohen. For me he was a father figure, a man who helped me find at least a little of the thing I cared about the most: understanding drug abuse. He died a few months after my own father died. That made his loss even more poignant for me. When I was given the opportunity to write this foreword I was delighted and grateful. Here was my chance to pay my respects to a valued mentor and to share his gift with a larger audience. Hopefully, his last book will reach a wider audience than those already familiar with Sidney Cohen's writing. In *The Chemical Brain*, Dr. Cohen takes the reader on a marvelous journey of discovery into a world he knew better than anyone else who ever passed that way.

Sidney Cohen, M.D., was the best writer in the drug abuse field during the last two decades. His ability to communicate the most sophisticated science in ways that were accessible to broad audiences was without peer. In *The Chemical Brain* we not only have his last book, but the book which summarized his vast learning in one volume of which he was uniquely proud. Here interested students of the brain, of behavior, and of drug dependence can all find a brilliant summary of the latest scientific knowledge. Sidney Cohen left us this legacy. Readers of this book will come to share my deeply personal sense of gratitude to him for his gift even as we mourn his passing.

This foreword is my gift to him. His book, *The Chemical Brain*, is his gift to all of us. We can best repay him by enjoying the pursuit of understanding of one of life's great questions: how the brain works. He enjoyed that pursuit every day of his life.

Robert L. DuPont, M.D.
Former Director, National Institute on Drug Abuse
Chairman, Center for Behavioral Medicine
Rockville, Maryland

Preface

The Chemical Brain is an attempt to fuse recent information and hypotheses about the biochemical processes involved in mental functioning. As recently as a dozen years ago little of what is written here was known or even imagined. Now we can discern a number of patterns of brain cell organization and function. Some of these ideas will require revision in the coming years. Nevertheless, it is important to be aware of the major increments in knowledge and technology that have occurred within a relatively brief period of time.

The emphasis here is on biochemistry, actually neurochemistry. This by no means denies the input of social, cultural and psychological elements in the productions of the brain. Indeed, it seems likely that these inputs also come to have chemical representation. This is certainly true in the chemistry of memory. But I am referring to something more: that the impacts of the sociocultural environment and of what we call mind certainly affect the chemical transactions that go on within the neurons—and they in turn, are affected by the neurochemical state.

On the autopsy table we see a three-pound, pink-gray, nondescript, gelatin-like mass. Except for a number of wrinkles and bulges, it could be something that has been prepared for eventual breadmaking. Its electrical production is trivial. Harnessing the entire central nervous system's electrical output could hardly light up a 20-watt bulb. Nonetheless, its capabilities transcend any known device, instrument or system.

In our exploration of the chemistry of this marvelous organ, a strenuous effort has been made to provide a second-level book, neither a primer for beginners nor a treatise for the researcher, rather a simpler volume for the health professional and for the lay person with some basic information or interest in biochemistry. A certain amount of technical language has been necessary, but explanations of such terms appear in the text or in the glossary. Many abbreviations are used because they are the jargon of science, but they are paired with the words from which they have been derived when first encountered and also are to be found in the glossary if recall fails.

As indicated, research on neurochemistry is in a state of flux. Although substantial changes in our understanding will be necessary eventually, this does not diminish the value of the data and concepts acquired in recent times. Without them, we remain in a sort of Dark Ages of understanding the nature of the brain. With them, we approach a Middle Age, and in the distance, we might perceive a brightening.

The reading I have done and conversations I have had while writing this book have led to some overall conclusions about the expanse of the brain. I offer these here because, while relevant to the chemistry of the brain, they go beyond it. I have acquired a new respect, indeed awe, for the potential of the brain, the dimensions of which are not yet visible. Here, then, are some of the properties of the brain that seem most impressive.

1. Flexibility

When we reflect upon the chemistry of the brain, it becomes impressive how flexible the system is. Its messages can be quite variable, not necessarily limited to "go" or "no go." Neurons can adapt to new internal and external situations. The brain has a remarkable capacity to review and renew its circuitry within hours. Even the death of adjacent cells can be compensated for by the extension of dendrites from surviving neurons, reestablishing the lost connections. The discovery that more than one transmitter can operate within a neuron, and that neurons may even change transmitters, adds to the multiplicity of options available. The brain is certainly no black box with a stimulus entering at one end and a response issuing from the other. Neither is the wiring diagram completely hardened, as was once thought.

2. Complexity

When complexity achieves a certain order of magnitude, function becomes unpredictable. What we know of the neuron, the basic unit, may not apply to billions of neurons with trillions of interconnections acting together. The brain has evidently achieved a level of intricacy that endows it with capabilities greater than the sum of its multitudinous parts. This provides the brain and its product, the mind, with superlative capabilities of consciousness, imagination, creativity, integrated thought, abstraction and correlational capabilities well beyond what could be predicted by studying the neuron.

3. Regulation

The degree of control and regulation over brain activity is quite astonishing. Equally striking is the ability of the cortex to override the automatic regulatory systems that, usually, work so well. A person may be starving with a low brain glucose level and with food available, yet the food will be ignored if certain ideas about the significance of the food dominate thought. People can be trained to control their blood pressure, heart rate and awareness of pain.

These and similar functions are regulated by set points. Core body temperatures, for example, are remarkably fixed, fluctuating within a degree of 98.6°F (37°C). Even the diurnal temperature fluctuations are strikingly predictable. The set point is fixed by a combination of neuroendocrine, central nervous system (CNS) and autonomic thermoreceptors. The temperature of the blood flowing through the hypothalamus and in the skin determines whether an increase or decrease in the core temperature should occur. Dilation of the small blood vessels in the skin and perspiration will cause heat loss. Constriction of the capillaries of the skin, shivering, and physical activity will produce heat gain. Temperature homeostasis results from the sum of these and other heat-regulating mechanisms—a remarkable accomplishment.

At the level of the neuron, the many controls over transmission seem almost redundant. A variety of ion fluxes can modify firing. Precursor availability and their enzyme systems determine whether and how much of the transmitter is released into the synapse. The catabolizing enzyme activity and the efficiency of transmitter reuptake also determine whether subsequent transmission will occur. Calcium ions (Ca^{++}) control discharge of transmitters into the synapse. Meanwhile, at the presynaptic terminal the message can be further modulated by neurohormones and neuropeptides. And this is not the end. At the receptor sites on the postsynaptic neuron a variety of changes can occur that may block or enhance further passage of the signal. Why this abundance of checks and balances?

4. Brain-Body Interactions

The CNS influences every body cell. The cerebral cortex and the subcortex, through thought and emotion, contribute to this influence. Innumerable examples of this psychosomatic relationship are available. The converse, the somatopsychic impact of body states upon mental processes, is also recognized. In certain areas information is incomplete, for example, the nature of the linkage between the brain function and the immune system. Can mental set affect resistance to infections and other immune diseases like malignancies?

One fairly obvious area of future inquiry is in the exposure to, and duration of, severe stress. Learned stress management techniques are capable of reducing our responses to inordinate stress. Prolonged, severe stress can alter the cortisol receptors in the hypothalamus, thereby eliminating the feedback circuit that ordinarily would turn off the stress response. Therefore, the reaction to stress will continue even in its absence, eventually producing the diseases of stress.

5. Detail and Replication

The enormous duplication of the CNS is impressive. Although memories are laid down on specific neurons, they may also be invoked by stimulating other brain areas. In young humans almost half a hemisphere can be removed without producing a critical disruption of mental functioning. Multiple pacemakers seem to exist for most rhythms of the brain. Up to a point, the brain will find a way.

6. Filtering

As noteworthy as any quality is the brain's ability to filter out the flood of incoming sensory information, allowing only the novel, the threatening, or focused information to come through to consciousness. Many thousand bits of information are simultaneously impinging on the brain from the sensory organs and memory stores. The vast majority of these are quenched, perhaps in the raphe and adjoining structures; otherwise we would be in a constant buzzing confusion. It may be that in certain psychotic states the filtering system is disrupted.

7. Organization

From what is known of the structural and functional organization of the brain, its development is a remarkable achievement. In the three-week embryo the brain is a fold of neural tissue. A week or two later it is a tube with bulges that will become its major subdivisions. A primitive eye is becoming visible. The embryonic brain goes through stages that recapitulate the brains of simpler animals.

How do the billions of nerve cells recognize each other and know where to migrate? How do the neural connections know which cells to connect to? Is it a hit-or-miss affair with unwanted synapses dying? Or are surface antigens already present to guide them? And the ultimate question: How does the brain develop the qualities we call mind and consciousness?

8. Survivability

The function of the brain is to process information about the external and internal environments, then to develop responses to these data. The responses may be to think or to act. On a less than conscious level the response may require a change to maintain homeostasis and preserve body equilibrium. Usually, but far from always, the responses are to increase chances of survival, directly or indirectly. These organismic responses in the direction of survival can be matched on a molecular level. DNA, the molecule from which all proteins and peptides flow, has its own specific repair enzymes that are apparently not used for other purposes. If DNA is damaged by carcinogens, a fair amount of repair is still possible. So for every cancer that becomes manifest, many are apparently avoided.

The brain is protected from some, but not all, toxins by a blood-brain barrier. Lipid soluble substances like alcohol, nicotine, heroin, and diazepam, readily pass into the brain. Water-soluble chemicals are selectively processed across a unique capillary endothelium into brain tissues. The barrier does not exist around the pituitary and pineal glands or at the hypothalamus. This is fortunate because it allows hormones providing feedback information from the rest of the body to reach these areas so that regulation of the neuroendocrine system can occur.

But there is a vast sphere of human existence that lies beyond survival. The brain has the propensity to develop abstract thoughts and concepts, art forms, and other nonsurvival-oriented activities. Wonder about the meaning of life is a perennial human inquiry apparently shared by few other species, if any. These extrasurvival mental productions may represent the thought sequences generated by the sheer complexity of the human brain.

To learn more about the nature of the brain is an end in itself. Further, an understanding of how mind- and mood-altering drugs impact upon it has become essential information for the mental health professional. The emphasis here is on the neurochemistry of the addictive disorders. It will surprise no one to find most of the psychotherapeutic drugs included within this category.

Using the first two chapters as a basis for understanding neuronal function, the subsequent chapters on the chemistry, the pharmacotherapy, and the genetics of addiction provide the mechanism of action for these drugs. A final chapter on brain imaging brings us up to date on the remarkable new techniques of perceiving the structure and function of the brain.

1

The Chemical Neuron

"No crooked thought without a crooked molecule."

At some level all brain cell activity is chemical. Even the conduction of signals along the neuronal membrane, although an electrical transmission, is based on chemical shifts across the membrane. The replication of the DNA molecular chain is chemically generated and controlled. The synthesis and delivery of neurotransmitters are, of course, biochemical events. The hormones generated within the brain, and those delivered to the central nervous system from other organs, all exert chemical effects. Likewise drugs, licit and illicit, act by influencing the brain's chemistry.

Some neuropsychiatric disorders are based upon structural errors or distortions. However, increasing numbers are evidently molecular or macromolecular aberrations and have become, or will be amenable to, corrective chemotherapies.

Many of the mind's functions like sleep and waking, memory, mood and affect, thought, perception and consciousness are beginning to be understood in terms of chemical transactions. We are only at the threshold of an understanding of what will be called psychoneurochemistry of mentation.

Anatomy of the Neuron

In order to understand neuronal function something about its structure should be recalled.

The Dendrites

These consist of hundreds or thousands of widely branched extensions that serve to receive impulses from the axons of other neurons by means of their receptor sites on the dendritic postsynaptic membrane. An action current then travels down the dendrite to the cell body and down the axon by ion transmission.

The Cell Body

The cell body (also soma or perikaryon) contains a number of important structures.

• The Nucleus

The nucleus contains the genetic material within chromosomes. It is encoded as long chains of DNA (deoxyribonucleic acid). The DNA sequence is transcribed to messenger RNA (mRNA), ribonucleic acid. mRNA moves into the cytoplasm, where it serves as a template upon which proteins and peptides are fabricated. The neuron is constantly renewing all of its proteins. Every 15 days a 90% turnover of cell protein takes place.

• The Endoplasmic Reticulum (Ribosomes)

The endoplasmic reticulum is a network of channels in the cytoplasm that provides for the transfer of materials down into the axon. It consists of a rough endoplasmic reticulum that synthesizes products needed for cell function. The smooth endoplasmic reticulum (Golgi apparatus) packages these products to prevent their enzymatic destruction while in transit down the axon.

The Axon

The axon is an elongated process ending in a terminal bouton that contacts one or usually more dendrites, translates their message into specific neurochemical transmitters, and delivers them into the synaptic microspace.

- The Microtubules

These thin structures deliver molecule-sized materials from the cell body to the terminal bouton. Precursors of transmitters and cell nutrients are moved in this manner. Retrograde transport also occurs.

- The Mitochondria

The mitochondria produce high-energy organic phosphates by synthesizing low energy phosphate molecules with oxygen and glucose. They are the energy generators for most chemical activities in the neuron.

- The Synaptic Vesicles

The synaptic vesicles are tiny sacs which store 1,000 to 50,000 molecules of a transmitter and, at the proper signal, eject them at the synaptic membrane. This process is called exocytosis. After the transmitter acts on the postsynaptic receptor site, reuptake by the vesicles occurs, protecting the transmitter from metabolizing enzymes either in the synaptic cleft or in the cytoplasm of the axon terminal. Reuptake by the vesicles is an active process that can be visualized as a molecular pump.

The Presynaptic Membrane

The entire cell membrane of the neuron acts as a mechanism for the movement of electrolytes (as ions), nutrients, water, the building blocks of a variety of peptides, phospholipids and proteins. In addition, unneeded chemicals are removed across the membrane into glial cells.

The membrane consists of an inner and outer surface made up of phospholipids, lipoproteins and glycoproteins in an aqueous substrate. Tiny ion channels that are specific for potassium (K^+), sodium (Na^+), chloride (Cl^-) and calcium (Ca^{++}) have been identified. They are capable of selectively opening and closing upon minute electrical or chemical commands. Other ion channels remain open at all times. The membrane glycoproteins and lipoproteins probably represent the receptor sites. They also surround the ion channel pores.

The presynaptic membrane of the axon terminal is distinctive in that it permits the discharge of neurotransmitters from the vesicles into the synaptic space. The vesicle fuses with the cell membrane before discharging its contents. Transmitter reuptake consists of reversing the process.

The Synapse

The synapse is a minute space that exists between the presynaptic axonal membrane of one neuron and the postsynaptic dendrite membrane of the receiving neurons. It contains the neurotransmitter molecules that will lock onto the receptor sites and the excess molecules that will not find a recognition site. Present in the synaptic space are enzymes that metabolize the free transmitter molecules unless they are quickly removed from the synapse.

FIGURE I

SCHEMATIZED NEURON

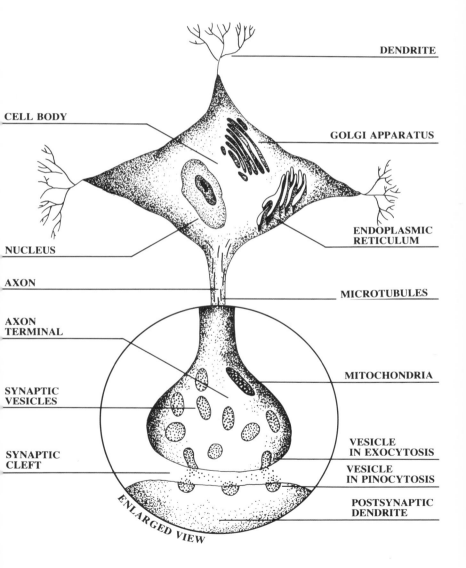

The Postsynaptic Membrane

This membrane is ordinarily on a dendrite of the neuron receiving the chemical information bit from the antecedent neuron. It contains the protein that is specially tailored in shape and electric charge to receive the transmitter.

The Autoreceptors

Autoreceptors are recognition sites on the presynaptic neuron. They receive feedback information from postsynaptic neurons about the level of receptor occupancy, thereby regulating subsequent transmitter release.

The Glia

In addition to the billions of nerve cells within the skull, even more glia cells are present. Glia makes up more than half the volume of the brain. It provides structural support of the neurons and is its supply system. Everything needed to form neurotransmitters and proteins is transferred: water, oxygen and glucose, and oxygen. Without them, the nerve cells start dying off within minutes because the brain has no capability to store glucose. Glucose is essentially the exclusive source of energy for its multitude of chemical transactions. In the resting state 20% of the body's oxygen intake is consumed by the brain. In a cascade of chemical reactions glucose and oxygen are almost entirely transformed to carbon dioxide and water.

Certain glia cells, the oligodendrocytes, wrap themselves around the neuronal axon providing a myelin sheath that insulates it and accelerates transmission of the electrochemical impulse. This is of great advantage when rapid responses are needed. Demyelinizing diseases like multiple sclerosis are caused by toxic, infectious, or autoimmune disorders of the myelin sheath.

Another glia cell type is the astrocyte. It forms an important part of the blood-brain barrier, preventing many molecules which could damage cell function from entering the brain. Even a small molecule like the transmitter dopamine is incapable of penetrating across the blood-brain barrier. Instead, its precursor, dihydroxyphenylalanine (dopa), passes into the glia, and then to neurons. The enzyme that converts dopa to dopamine, dopamine decarboxylase, is synthesized in the cell body and then is transported to the axon terminal, where the synthesis to dopamine takes place. After the discharge of a neurotransmitter into the synapse, glia cells are capable of taking up some of the excess neurotransmitter molecules. This avoids their breakdown by catabolizing enzymes in the synapse. The glia cells transfer the transmitter back into the neuron.

Electrochemistry of the Neuron

The discovery that chemicals are involved in the nerve cell transmission process is not old. Sixty-five years ago Otto Loewi proved that a specific chemical agent which he called "parasympathin" was manufactured by stimulating a cranial nerve, the vagus, and that it caused a slowing of the heart rate. That substance is now called acetylcholine. It would take three more decades before the chemical mediation of central synaptic transmission was established. The first edition of Goodman and Gilman's *Pharmacological Basis of Therapeutics* (1941) could only say: "The evidence for the role of a chemical mediator in central transmission is, as yet, meager."

About 60 substances are now known to have CNS effects as neurotransmitters, neuromodulators, and mediators of neuronal function. It is estimated that eventually some 300 endogenous chemicals with CNS activity will be identified.

The brain contains about a hundred billion neurons, and some neurons receive information from hundreds to thousands of its connections, the dendrites. This complexity of signals ordinarily passes down single axons to a terminal where it connects with dendrites from other neurons across a microscopic space, the synapse. The synaptic cleft is one of the crucial decision points where the presynaptic transmitting neuron discharges molecules into the synapse to be moved onto the postsynaptic (receiving) neuron's receptor sites that are specifically shaped for that transmitter's molecule. No chemical fit, no message. But it is not the single neuronal event that counts. Neuronal clusters acting in unison reinforce or quench the information bits at the postsynaptic recognition (receptor) site. It is reasonable to think of the brain as a symphony of almost infinite orchestration with assemblies of instrumentations evoking an infinite ensemble of informational responses. The brain, vast and adaptable, is capable of providing for all the subtleties of sensing, integrating and responding.

The brain not only talks to itself in an array of chemical languages, but it also answers back. It is also listening to the sensory flood out there—the unending signals of perception—and in here—the selectively retrieved memories. Meanwhile, the condition of its landlord, the body, is monitored by feedback messages delivered by the blood and the autonomic or peripheral nerves. Only after reducing and fusing this cascade of information are the final decisions called "behavior," in the broad sense of the word, executed.

The neuron is the basic information processor and transmitter. Conduction is an electrical phenomenon based upon membrane potential changes that depend on voltage differences between intracellular and extracellular ions. The presence of high intracellular and low extracellular potassium (K^+) ions produces a negative charge with a resting membrane potential of -70 mV (millivolts). At this point the membrane is polarized (charged).

Depolarization (or discharge) occurs when sodium (Na^+) channels are opened in the membrane, reducing the voltage difference to below -35 mV. As the voltage differential falls, an action potential is generated. Depolarization progresses as more sodium channels synchronously open along the route of the dendrite, past the cell body and down the axon. The sodium surge is excitatory. The entry of sodium ions into the cell during depolarization produces a flow of potassium ions out of the cell that lasts 1 msec (millisecond). Near the cell body, if chloride (Cl^-) channels are opened, the negative voltage will increase to -90 mV, depolarization is inhibited, and the action current is quenched. The membrane is hyperpolarized (refractory).

The neuronal membrane is negatively charged because the negative chloride, carbonate, and phosphate ions inside the cells are present in amounts greater than the positive intracellular potassium. An ion pump forces sodium ions out of the neuron as K^+, water and sugar enter, adding to the negative charge within the cell.

When the action potential arrives near the presynaptic terminal, calcium (Ca^{++}) ion channels open, and a calcium flux into the cell occurs. This triggers the release of the neurotransmitter for 1 to 2 msec. The presence of large numbers of calcium ions in the terminal bouton produces a further release of transmitter for about a second (slow type transmission). The total amount of transmitter release is proportional to the amount of intracellular calcium. In a calcium-free medium, no transmitter release occurs. If the calcium available is increased, more transmitter is released. Therefore, calcium channel blockers will inhibit the transmission of the impulse.

In the periphery, the smooth muscles, for example, do not contract when Ca^{++} antagonists are introduced. The antidiarrheal effects of diphenoxylate (Lomotil) are, in part, due to a Ca^{++} channel blockade. Opioids in general tend to block the Ca^{++} release of transmitters and many of their functions are understandable on this basis. Calcium ion flux inhibitors that do not pass the blood-brain barrier, like veropamil (Calan, Isoptin), relax coronary artery spasm, and reduce oxygen utilization by lowering arterial pressure and by dilating the peripheral arterioles. They are useful in angina, hypertension and certain arrythmias.

Central nervous system Ca^{++} ion flux inhibitors (nimodipine) are becoming available and act to inhibit neuronal transmission, thereby preventing paroxysmal depolarization and seizure activity. Ca^{++} enters the neuron by combining with calmodulin, a Ca^{++} receptor protein, which regulates the degree of phosphorylation and thereby regulates the release of neurotransmitters. The Ca^{++} ion is necessary for the induction of seizures; therefore, a new class of anticonvulsants may become available—the central Ca^{++} channel blockers. Calcium channel blockers have also been used as antimigraine and antimanic drugs.

This brief story of CNS ion transmission is told because it is a fundamental characteristic of neuronal tissue. The ion flux along the membrane is propagated in rapid wavelike sequences. Interferences with neuronal transmission induce derangements which will be discussed.

2

Neurotransmitters, Neuropeptides and Neurohormones

It may be that most neurons contain multiple transmitters, for example, an amine or amino acid, along with a neuropeptide to modulate the transmission and sometimes a neurohormone to prolong the transmission. All neurochemical information circuits are widely dispersed and are almost never localized in discrete brain areas. As a corollary, many neurotransmitting systems converge on single brain regions. These features of transmitter function make simple statements about the effects of various transmitters incomplete. Furthermore, the receptors exhibit a considerable self-regulatory capability, changing their sensitivity during excessive or infrequent use.

Many of the important transmitters are amines and are called biogenic amines as a group. Most are monoamines; that is, they have a single ammonium (NH_2) radical in their structure. The biogenic amines derived from catechol (dihydrobenzene) are named catecholamines and include dopamine, norepinephrine, and epinephrine. Another monoamine is serotonin, 5-hydroxytryptamine. Acetylcholine is not an amine. It does not contain an NH_2 group. It can be classified as a choline ester.

Neurotransmitters

Acetylcholine (ACh)

The cholinergic (ACh) system can be understood as a portion of the brain's and body's quiet attention and preparation for

TABLE I
SOME PRESUMPTIVE NEUROTRANSMITTERS

Class	Name, Abbreviation	Receptor Subtypes	Synthesizing Enzyme	Catabolizing Enzyme	Agonist	Antagonist	Action
Choline esters	Acetylcholine (ACh)	M_1 M_2 N	Choline Acetyltranferase	Acetylcholine esterase	Muscarine (M) Nicotine (N)	Atropine Curare	M_1 Excitatory M_2 Inhibitory N Excitatory
Monoamines	Dopamine (DA)	D_1 D_2 D_3 D_4	Dopa Dicarboxylase	MAO COMT	Bromocriptine Apomorphine	Phenothiazine Haloperidol	Inhibitory
	Norepinephrine (NE)	a_1 a_2 b_1 b_2	Dopamine beta Hydroxylase	MAO COMT	a_1 Phenylephrine a_2 Clonidine b_1 Dobutamine	a_1 Prazosin a_2 Yohinbine b_1 Propranolol	Inhibitory
	Epinephrine (E)		Norepinephrine N-methyltransferase	MAO COMT	Similar to NE		Inhibitory
	Serotonin (5-HT)	5-HT 5-HT	Tryptophan Decarboxylase	MAO COMT	LSD	Methysergide	Inhibitory
	Histamine (H)	H_1 H_2	Histidine Decarboxylase	MAO	H_1 Betahistine H_2 Betazole	H_1 Pyrilamine H_2 Cimetidine	Excitatory Inhibitory
Amino acids:	Gamma amino butyric acid (GABA)	GABA-A GABA-B	Glutamic acid Decarboxylase	GABA-transaminase	A Muscimol B Baclofen	A Picrotoxin B Bicuculine	Inhibitory
	Glycine		Serine trans-hydroxymethylase		Beta alanine	Strychnine	Inhibitory
	Glutamate		Glutaminases	Glutamine synthesase	Kainic acid	Glutamate diethylester	Excitatory
Purines	Adenosine	P_1					Inhibitory
	Adenosine triphosphate	P_2					Inhibitory
Neuropeptides	See Table II						

action. ACh neurons respond to messages from the internal and external environment and deliver an integrated physiologic and behavioral response.

Cholinergic mechanisms are responsible, in part, for conservation of energy, attention, memory, defense or aggression, thirst, sexual behavior, mood, play and REM sleep. Much of the brain's ACh is produced in the basal forebrain and extends to other brain areas. Cholinergic neurons are found in the hippocampus and the cortex, participating in learning, memory formation, and retrieval.

Parasympathetic stimulation (ACh neurons in the autonomic nervous system to the viscera) slows the heart, reduces blood pressure, increases gastrointestinal activity, constricts the pupils and the bronchial tubes, and empties the bladder and rectum. These visceral functions are activated by muscarinic ACh neurons and act on muscarinic receptors. Muscarine itself is an ACh agonist. Atropine blocks muscarinic activity and produces opposing glandular and smooth muscle effects to those mentioned above.

Nicotinic ACh fibers act on striated (skeletal) muscles, and nicotine mimics their effects. Muscle contraction is the result. The nicotinic receptor has been isolated and its structure is known. Curare is a nicotinic antagonist, and it paralyzes skeletal muscles. Botulin, the active component of botulism poison, blocks the release of ACh at both nicotinic and muscarinic receptors.

Acetylcholine is synthesized at the terminal axon by combining choline with acetyl coenzyme A in the presence of the enzyme choline acetyltransferase. ACh is eventually metabolized by acetylcholinesterase to choline and acetic acid. The choline is taken up into the presynaptic neuron for reuse.

Anticholinesterases, as would be expected, prolong ACh action and are capable of causing convulsions and death. They act upon both nicotinic and muscarinic neurons. Physostigmine from the African Calabar or ordeal bean is the traditional anticholinesterase inhibitor and is effective in treating atropine poisoning. Malathion and other insecticides and certain nerve gases are irreversible anticholinesterases and, for that reason, are highly toxic. Physostigmine and pilocarpine have been used to constrict the pupils in the treatment of glaucoma.

Anticholinergic drugs are widely represented in therapeutics. Atropine and its antecedent, belladonna, have been long known for their anticholinergic autonomic activity. Antispasmotics, anti-Parkinsonian agents, neuroleptics, antidepressants, many pupillary dilators, and some preoperative medications (to dry oral secretions) have anticholinergic activity. Scopolamine induces a drowsy euphoria and amnesia (once used in obstetrics as twilight sleep) because of its greater degree of central anticholinergic effect than atropine.

A balance between cholinergic and dopaminergic activity exists in the basal ganglia to control muscle tone, fine movements, and posture. When more than 80% of the dopaminergic fibers are destroyed, Parkinsonism results. It can be treated by loading with L-dopa, a precursor of dopamine, or by giving a dopamine agonist like bromocriptine (Parlodel). Alternatively, anticholinergic agents like benztropine (Cogentin) will also reduce the tremor and rigidity of Parkinsonism by blocking cholinergic receptors and reducing the cholinergic preponderance over dopaminergic activity in the extrapyramidal nuclei.

Myasthenia gravis is an autoimmune disease caused by the development of antibodies to the nicotinic receptor protein, resulting in loss of most receptor sites in the skeletal muscles. It is marked by easy fatigability and generalized weakness similar to curare poisoning. Dramatic improvement occurs with an anticholinesterase like neostigmine (Prostigmin).

Dementia of the Alzheimer Type (DAT)

In addition to the structural changes (senile plaques, neurofi-

brillary tangles, and cortical atrophy), some chemical alterations have been consistently documented in DAT. A decrease
in choline acetyltransferase, the enzyme that makes ACh, is
found. ACh neuronal loss also occurs, so that cholinergic
mechanisms tend to be severely reduced in DAT. Drugs that
block muscarinic receptors (scopolamine, atropine), when
given to normal young adults, reproduce a number of the cognitive defects of early DAT. Such agents will also worsen the
disease. Although the central cholinergic system is distinctly
disrupted, noradrenergic pathways in the locus ceruleus (blue
spot) also manifest substantial cell loss. Dementias of Down's
syndrome and Parkinsonism also are accompanied by a reduction of cholinergic activity.

Alzheimer's disease is presumed to be, at least in part, a
deficiency of cholinergic neurons in the forebrain. Transient
improvement has occurred with physostigmine therapy. What
is needed for therapeutic efficacy is long-acting, highly
specific cholinomimetic agents of low toxicity. Tetrahy-
droaminoacridine (THA), a cholinesterase inhibitor, is now
being evaluated in DAT patients. The forebrain cholinergic
circuits are involved in the transfer of recent memory to permanent memory stores; thus their absence contributes to the
memory deficiency of Alzheimer's disease.

A group of diseases characterized by both movement disorders and dementia includes Huntington's chorea, Fried-
reich's ataxia and Gilles de la Tourette's disease, and they
may be associated with ACh deficiency. Therefore choline has
been recommended with variable success. No evidence exists
that ingested choline increases ACh levels in the brain. Antipsychotic drugs, particularly haloperidol (Haldol), are used to
provide dopamine blockade for the neurologic and the psychiatric aspects of these conditions and to reduce the ACh/DA
imbalance.

Mood changes caused by shifts in cholinergic activity
have been reported: decreased activity evokes euphoria, and

increased activity produces a depressive state.

A nerve growth factor (NGF) previously found only in peripheral nerves has been recovered in brain neurons, particularly in cholinergic neurons. NGF is necessary for the development and maintenance of ACh mediated neurons, including those involved in memory.

Catecholamines

The catecholamines include dopamine, norepinephrine and epinephrine. Their precursor is the amino acid, tyrosine, which is enzymatically transformed into the various catecholamines. The transformation from tyrosine to one of the three catecholamines is shown in Figure II.

Alpha methyltyrosine blocks the synthesis of all catecholamines, particularly norepinephrine, by inhibiting the enzyme tyrosine hydroxylase; this is the rate-limiting step.

Dopamine (DA)

The essential action of DA is to respond with appetitive and reward-seeking (reinforcing) behaviors. These pleasure-driven responses might tempt one to call dopamine the "gusto" transmitter. Sensory, motor, and neurohormonal activities process the motivated approach behaviors. Some of dopamine's principle activities include:

1. Neurons in the substantia nigra (the black substance) manufacture DA for delivery to the caudate nucleus of the basal ganglia. Fine movements and muscle tone are under control of this region. A marked decrease or absence of DA (particularly the D_2 receptors) is found in Parkinsonism. DA loss contributes to depressive psychoses.

FIGURE II

CATECHOLAMINE PATHWAYS

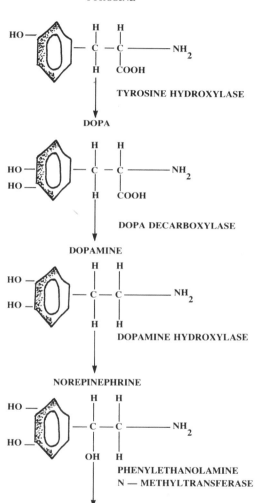

TYROSINE

TYROSINE HYDROXYLASE

DOPA

DOPA DECARBOXYLASE

DOPAMINE

DOPAMINE HYDROXYLASE

NOREPINEPHRINE

PHENYLETHANOLAMINE
N — METHYLTRANSFERASE

EPINEPHRINE

2. Dopaminergic neurons extend from the ventral tegmentum in the midbrain to the part of the limbic system concerned with emotionality and reward. Another bundle of DA neurons proceeds to the frontal cortex where thoughts and emotions are integrated. An increased sensitivity of DA receptors in this system is associated with the schizophrenic syndrome. This is the rationale of the treatment of schizophrenia with dopamine blockers like the phenothiazines (e.g., Thorazine), the butyrophenones (e.g., Haldol) and the thioxanthines (e.g., Navane). These neuroleptics can induce Parkinsonism because the blockade also affects dopamine transmission in the basal ganglia. Anticholinergic drugs effectively correct this complication of the neuroleptics by reducing the DA/ACh imbalance. (See Fig. III.)

Some psychotic patients require antipsychotic medication for years, producing a prolonged DA blockade. This may result in DA basal ganglia receptor hypersensitivity because increased numbers of receptors had formed (upregulation). Now, ordinary amounts of dopamine cause dopaminergic overactivity. A movement disorder, tardive dyskinesia, marked by involuntary rhythmic tongue, jaw, head and other body movements, can emerge. Normally, tardive dyskinesia is observed after the neuroleptic has been decreased or stopped. At this point, the dopamine blockade is reduced, and the patient's ordinary DA production causes DA hypersensitivity and tardive dyskinesia, a difficult condition to treat.

FIGURE III

DA/ACh STRIATAL INTERACTIONS

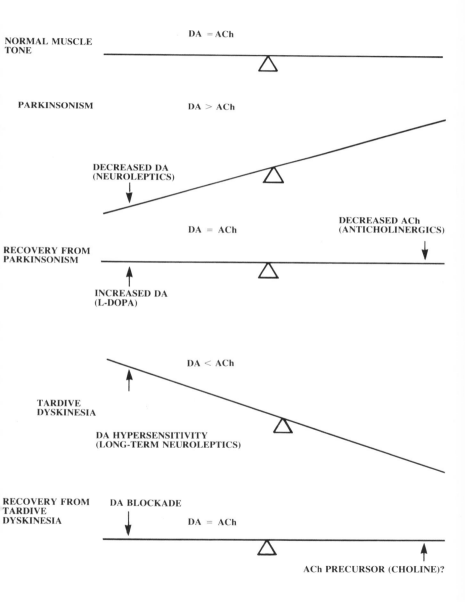

3. Coming from the cortex and midbrain, dopaminergic neurons stimulate hypothalamic discharge of releasing hormones that generate the production of thyrotropic, gonadotropic and adrenocorticotropic hormones. Prolactin release is inhibited by dopamine; therefore, neuroleptics increase it. Galactorrhea, abnormal milk secretion, is sometimes a side effect of neuroleptic therapy.

Dopamine serves as a good example of how drugs can impact on the activity of biogenic amines.

1. Decrease of dopaminergic activity:

• Alpha methyltyrosine (no therapeutic use).

• Alpha methyldopa (Aldomet) inhibits the enzyme dopa decarboxylase that transforms dopa to DA, thereby decreasing its availability. Aldomet is an antihypertensive agent.

• Reserpine (Serpasil) induces a release of DA from the protective vesicles in the axon into the cytoplasm where it can be metabolized by monoamine oxidase (MAO). It has been of some use as an antihypertensive and antipsychotic agent. Monoamine oxidase inhibitors (MAOIs) will neutralize the effects of MAO.

• All neuroleptics block dopamine receptor sites by competitively inhibiting the activation of the enzyme adenylate cyclase, thus decreasing the amount of the second messenger, cAMP, (cyclic adenosine monophosphate).

• The antiemetic effects of neuroleptics like

prochlorperazine (Compazine) are due to their blocking action of DA receptors in the chemoreceptor trigger zone in the emetic center of the medulla. Apomorphine and other dopamine agonists often produce vomiting. They have been used in aversion treatment of alcoholism. Neuroleptics can prevent apomorphine-induced emesis according to their affinity for the dopamine binding sites in the emetic center.

2. Increase of dopaminergic activity:

• L-dopa therapy for Parkinsonism increases the synthesis of DA by increasing precursor availability.

• CNS euphorostimulants like cocaine, amphetamines, and methylphenidate (Ritalin) encourage the release of monoamines, including DA, and prevent their reuptake back into the presynaptic neuronal vesicles. Thus by increased DA availability in the synapse initially, they serve as a model of schizophrenia in large doses. The CNS stimulants may also exacerbate schizophrenic symptoms or cause a relapse in a schizophrenic in remission.

• MAOIs like phenelzine (Nardil) prevent monoamine oxidase from degrading DA. MAOIs are antidepressants and antihypertensives.

• Bromocriptine (Parlodel) and amantidine (Symmetrel) activate postsynaptic dopamine receptors, thus inhibiting prolactin secretion, suppressing lactation, and reducing the dopamine deficiency in Parkinson's disease. It is being used to alleviate the dopamine deficiency of long-term cocaine consumption.

• Apomorphine is a dopamine agonist. It stimulates dopamine receptors in the corpus striatum, causing stereotyped movements (amphetamines and cocaine do likewise by other mechanisms). The differing ability of the neuroleptics to block apomorphine-induced stereotyped behavior predicts their potency as antipsychotic agents.

Schizophrenia

A considerable body of evidence suggests that schizophrenia is associated with dopamine overactivity or, what is more likely, a sensitization of dopamine receptors. Since dopamine turnover is not increased, it is probable that the postsynaptic receptor sites are hypersensitive to ordinary amounts of DA. Schizophrenics have an increased number of DA binding sites.

It has been shown that Type I schizophrenics, a syndrome associated with hallucinations, delusions, and overactivity, have increased numbers of DA_2 receptors. Type II schizophrenics, manifested by flattened affect, regression, withdrawal and, at times, cerebral atrophy, have no DA_2 receptor increase. It is likely that Type I schizophrenia is an early phase of the disorder, and that by the time that Type II symptoms appear, the dopamine receptor disturbance has subsided, and chronic residual symptoms remain. The drugs that are used in the treatment of the schizophrenic syndrome are more effective for the Type I disorder. All neuroleptics bind to the DA receptor, blockading postsynaptic transmission. Reserpine, which once was used for schizophrenia, depletes dopamine by preventing its entrance into the vesicles that protect it from the enzyme monoamine oxidase (MAO) in the cytoplasm.

Since the neuroleptics are so widely used in the treatment of schizophrenia and other psychoses, it may be well to describe additional side effects in terms of the neurochemical changes they produce.

In addition to blocking DA receptors, neuroleptics also block NE receptors. This can result in orthostatic (postural) hypotension and sedation. Haloperidol has a lower incidence of orthostatic hypotension and sedation than chlorpromazine because it produces less of an NE receptor blockade.

Parkinsonism (also the Extrapyramidal Syndrome, EPS)

In addition to what has already been said about Parkinsonism, some additional comments are appropriate. Idiopathic (of unknown origin), Parkinson's disease is usually a disorder of aging manifested by a rhythmic tremor of the hands and other areas, drooling, cogwheel rigidity, loss of spontaneous and associated movements, a blank stare, and a stooped posture. Parkinsonism is caused by the gradual loss of DA neurons over a lifetime until less than 20% remains. It may be that some as yet unidentified environmental toxin contributes to the dopaminergic depletion in the melanin-containing nigral cells. Carbon monoxide poisoning sometimes causes Parkinsonism. During the influenza epidemic of 1919-1920, thousands of people, young and old, developed an encephalitis that destroyed DA-producing cells and resulted in Parkinson's disease.

Another neurotoxin that destroys DA cells in the substantia nigra is 6-hydroxydopamine. The depletion of dopamine produces upregulation and an increase in the number of dopamine receptors on the postsynaptic membrane. There is evidence that chronic, high-dose amphetamine and methamphetamine use causes a metabolic diversion that produces 6-

hydroxydopamine. Whether long-term use of amphetamines will predispose people to Parkinsonism in later life is unknown.

A designer drug (a new analogue of an abused drug that produces similar effects) arrived on the street in 1984 and caused dozens of cases of acute, fulminating, irreversible Parkinsonism. An underground chemist wanted to synthesize a narcotic, MPPP. However, the synthesis was flawed and a related chemical, MPTP, was formed. This was sold as synthetic heroin and found its way into the veins of a few hundred people. As little as a single dose caused severe Parkinsonism in some users. MPTP is not the cause of the DA cell destruction. Instead, it is converted to MPP^+ by MAO in glial cells. MPP^+ selectively binds to neuromelanin contained in the substantia nigra with subsequent destruction of the DA neurons.

It has been found that older animals are more sensitive to MPTP than younger animals in their vulnerability to developing Parkinsonism. It may be that older animals have already lost many nigral DA cells in the course of aging, as all people do, and MPTP knocks out enough to cause clinical Parkinsonism. An alternative explanation may be that the increased MAO levels found in aging organisms permit a more ready conversion of MPTP to MPP^+.

One class of antipsychotic drugs exemplified by thioridazine (Mellaril) has a lower rate of extrapyramidal effects like tremor and muscle rigidity. Thioridazine has anticholinergic activity, reducing ACh at the same time that DA is lowered. When both transmitters are lowered, the Parkinsonism may not occur because it is the DA/ACh ratio of activity, not the level of DA or ACh, that produces Parkinsonism. High potency neuroleptics like trifluoperazine (Stelazine) and haloperidol (Haldol) have a much lower affinity for the muscarinic ACh receptor; therefore, the extrapyramidal syndrome (EPS) is more frequent with drugs of these types. A more recent theory of why a drug like thioridazine has a lower prevalence of Parkinsonism is that its DA blockade in the striatum is less intense than in the limbic system where its antipsychotic action is exerted.

As stated, the treatment of the EPS can be achieved by two measures: increasing dopamine levels in the striatum, or decreasing ACh in the same area. Decarboxylation of L-dopa provides dopamine. Most of the decarboxylation occurs in nonbrain tissues; therefore, the administration of a peripheral dopa decarboxyase inhibitor (carbidopa, Sinemet) permits a substantial decrease in the amount of L-dopa required to treat Parkinsonism.

Other dopaminergic tracts are affected by L-dopa, for example, the hypothalamic-pituitary axis, which affects hormonal secretion. Dopamine reduces prolactin secretion, and L-dopa does likewise.

Amantidine (Symmetrel), an antiviral agent, has a partial ameliorating effect on the EPS, because it facilitates the release of whatever dopamine remains in the presynaptic terminals.

Bromocriptine (Parlodel) is a dopamine (D_2) agonist that is useful in Parkinsonism. It is often used with L-dopa to prevent the "on-off" periods of ineffectiveness interspersed with periods of effectiveness of the latter drug.

Preliminary work with the grafting of dopamine-producing fetal brain cells or cells from the adrenal medulla has produced a temporary improvement in patients with the EPS. A considerable amount of work will be required before it is accepted as a viable treatment for Parkinsonism.

Norepinephrine (NE)

The noradrenergic transmitter, NE, produces an alerting, attention focusing, orienting response. Sensory arousal and motor and autonomic priming for "fight or flight" occur. Many waking activities like learning, memory, and awareness are mobilized by NE. In a sense NE is a serotonin antagonist.

NE is the sympathomimetic transmitter of the autonomic nervous system. It dilates the pupil, increases heart rate and blood pressure, constricts most arteries, and decreases gastrointestinal activity. Blood glucose rises and the bronchial tubes dilate. Skeletal muscle tone increases. These changes are advantageous for imminent action.

NE synthesis and breakdown is approximately similar to its precursor, dopamine. The major metabolic product of NE is MHPG (3-methoxy-4-hydroxyphenylglycol). It can be found in urine in decreased quantities in some depressive states, such as bipolar depression. Increases in urinary and plasma MHPG are often found in mania.

Three types of noradrenergic receptors exist. Alpha receptors are blockaded by phenoxybenzamine (Dibenzyline), which is used to control the hypertension and sweating that occurs with a pheochromocytoma. $Beta_1$ and $_2$ receptors are blocked by propranolol (Inderal), reducing heart rate, blood pressure, and cardiac output. $Beta_1$ receptors can be stimulated by dobutamine (Dobutrex) to increase contractions of the heart. $Beta_2$ agonists such as terbutaline (Brethine) can dilate the bronchioli without significant cardiac effects.

NE fibers can be found in all parts of the brain, but they constitute only one percent of the total transmitter content. Half of the NE-produced activation originates in the locus ceruleus and the lateral tegmentum. NE is distributed widely to induce a general level of arousal and excitability. NE also participates in learning and memory retrieval.

The monoaminergic theory of affective disorders is currently believed to be plausible. Much of the support for the belief that the monoamine transmitters have a central role in the genesis, and therefore the treatment, of affective disorders has arisen from clinical observations. These observations were later confirmed by animal and human research, namely:

1. Reserpine, which depletes the level of monoamines, can cause depression.

2. Monoamine oxidase inhibitors (MAOIs) elevate NE and serotonin (5-HT) availability and have an ameliorating effect on depressive moods.

3. Amphetamines and cocaine increase NE, DA, and 5-HT availability and have a temporary effect on depressive moods.

4. NE and 5-HT levels are lowered in depression. NE concentrations are elevated in mania.

5. Tricyclic antidepressants (TCAs) prevent the reuptake of NE and 5-HT, increasing their availability at receptor binding sites.

Two types of TCAs are identified. The tertiary amines, imipramine (Tofranil) and amitriptyline (Elavil), primarily block the reuptake of serotonin. The secondary amines, desipramine (Norpramin) and nortriptyline (Pamelor), block norepinephrine reuptake preferentially.

Not consistent with the monoaminergic theory is that the onset of action of TCAs is delayed for weeks despite the rapid availability of NE and 5-HT. Further, some antidepressants seem to have no effect upon monoamine reuptake. Lithium, helpful in bipolar disease, has only a modest effect on NE and 5-HT availability. Its major impact is upon cyclic adenosine monophosphate (cAMP) and the second messenger system.

At times patients who do not respond to one class of antidepressants may improve on an antidepressant of the other group.

TCAs are potent antihistamines because of their ability to block histamine (H_1) receptors. This accounts for the sedative property of antidepressants like amitriptyline and doxepin (Sinequan) and their additive effect with alcohol and other CNS depressants. In addition to their effects on the reuptake of NE, TCAs, particularly the tertiary amines, have an affinity for alpha-adrenergic receptors. This accounts for the decreased agitation, the tachycardia, and the hypotensive effects of these drugs. Blurred vision, dry mouth, urinary retention, constipation, and accelerated heart rhythm are due to a blockade of muscarinic receptors.

TCAs given over a period of weeks or months will increase NE availability with a secondary decrease in adrenoreceptors (downregulation). Monoamine oxidase inhibitors (MAOIs) produce the same effects, as does electroconvulsive therapy and REM sleep deprivation. These drugs and procedures have some antidepressant activity.

In major depressive disorders with a biogenic amine dysregulation there are secondary effects upon cortisol regulation. Hypothalamic-pituitary-adrenal cortex overactivity results in a hypersecretion of cortisol and a change in the circadian rhythm of cortisol secretion. Because of high levels of cortisol (depression may be stress-producing) depressed patients tend not to suppress cortisol secretion after 1 to 2 mg of dexamethasone. In nondepressed individuals, dexamethasone will block secretion of adrenocorticotrophic hormone (ACTH) because dexamethasone is perceived as cortisol. This provides a negative feedback signal to cortisol releasing factor and ACTH. The pituitary will decrease its secretion of ACTH, and cortisol production in the adrenals will be reduced.

The dexamethasone suppression test will reveal that 30 to 60% of major depressives will have a cortisol level above 5 mg/dl on the following day when dexamethasone was given at 11:00 P.M. the evening before. In other words, cortisol secretions were not suppressed, and the test was positive. With clinical improvement the test becomes negative.

Epinephrine (E) (Adrenaline)

The major function of epinephrine is at the periphery as a hormone secreted by the adrenal medulla. Recently, it was found in the CNS as a neurotransmitter located in the reticular formation. Its synthesis is from norepinephrine by methylation of the amine group by methyltransferase. The function of epinephrine in the brain is not yet clarified, although it could have a general activating function and affect blood pressure and respiratory rate.

Serotonin (5-HT, 5-hydroxytryptamine)

The amino acid, tryptophan, is converted by the enzyme, tryptophan hydoxylase, to 5-hydroxytryptophan, which is then transformed by tryptophan decarboxylase to 5-hydroxytryptamine, or serotonin. This is analogous to the process that converts tyrosine to dopamine. 5-HT is eventually oxidized to the inactive metabolite, 5-hydroxyindoleacetic acid (5-HIAA) and excreted in the urine, apparently in low levels in suicidal depressives.

Serotonin is an inhibitor of activity and behavior. It increases sleep time and reduces feeding, aggression, play and sexual activity. As suggested, 5-HT seems to be opposite to NE in its effects.

Most of the brain's serotonergic (also called tryptaminergic) cells are located in the raphe of the brain stem. Temperature regulation, sleep cycling, and to a certain extent, pain perception and mood states are attributed to 5-HT activity. Like dopamine, 5-HT participates in the production of the hypothalamic releasing hormones.

Large loading doses of the precursor tryptophan can increase 5-HT levels. The conversion of tryptophan to serotonin utilizes only about 1% of ingested tryptophan. The bulk of the amino acid is synthesized into protein. It cannot be expected that the amounts in certain foods, even when consumed in excess, will increase serotonergic firing. In fact, large amounts of presynaptic 5-HT will suppress such firing. It is occasionally used to procure sleep. The TCAs retard the reuptake of all biogenic amines and with some selectivity prevent 5-HT from returning to the presynaptic vesicles. Reserpine depletes 5-HT stores by releasing it from its storage sites in the vesicle along with other monoamines. Fenfluramine (Pondimin), although a sympathomimetic amine, depletes 5-HT levels, and therefore acts as an appetite reducer which sedates rather than stimulates. The MAOIs will inhibit the breakdown of 5-HT and increase its availability. Toxic agents that destroy serotonin-producing cells like 5-6-dihydroxytryptamine, MDA (methylene dioxyamphetamine, the Love Drug), and MDMA (methylenedioxymethylamphetamine, Ecstasy) are becoming known.

Serotonin serves as a precursor to the pineal gland hormone, melatonin, following stimulation of melanocyte-releasing hormone in the pituitary. The pineal gland contains large concentrations of 5-HT for conversion to melatonin, which plays a role in circadian rhythm changes, some depressions, light-dark cycles, the female reproductive cycle, jet lag and seasonal skin pigmentation changes. Seasonal variations in 5-HT levels have also been detected.

Life cycles retain an importance in CNS function despite our general unawareness of them and our attempts to defy them by moving across time zones, manipulating the menstrual cycle, and working night shifts. A science of chronopharmacology, the study of biochemicals that impact on life rhythms, is evolving. The pacemaker of the circadian rhythm (equal to a total cycle or lunar day, of 24.8 hours) is acetyltransferase, the enzyme that begins the conversion of 5-HT to melatonin. It is light sensitive, with larger amounts available during the day and lesser amounts at night. Diurnal changes in body temperature, sleep-wake cycles and the secre-

tion of pituitary hormones are regulated by melatonin, serotonin and other neurochemicals. The posterior pituitary hormone, vasopressin, is rhythmically discharged so that less
urine is secreted at night. ACTH from the anterior pituitary is
secreted in large amounts at dawn. It stimulates the production
of cortisol from the adrenal cortex, apparently to prepare the
body for the day's activity. Cognitive and psychomotor performance also correspond to rhythmic daily changes.

Lunar cycles have powerful impacts, especially upon the
female sex hormones whose production is controlled by
hypothalamic gonadotropin releasing hormones. Ovulation
and menstruation are supradiem (longer than a day) rhythms
that tend to be synchronous with the lunar phases. Hibernating
and migratory rhythms, which are probably genetically prog-
rammed, but are triggered by change in ambient temperature
and light, extend over many months. Mating rhythms, vestig-
ial in humans, are another example of supradiem clock.
"Winter depression" diagnosed in some people in temperate
and arctic zones may be caused by maladaptive responses to
extended dark periods and may be 5-HT-mediated. This seasonal depressive disorder is being treated with bright artificial
light.

The long sought after "s" (sleep) substance has not been
found, but a few facts are available. The activity of NE cells
in the locus ceruleus are maximal during awakening and alert-
ness. A slowing of locus ceruleus activity allows sleep to
begin. Serotonin is important in the sleep-wake cycle. Decreased 5-HT levels prevent sleep onset and diminish sleep
time. GABA (gamma aminobutyric acid) must also be involved in sleep, since it is the major inhibitor of excitatory
neurons in the brain.

Sleep itself is a complex activity with a rapid eye movement (REM) component and four types of non-REM sleep.
REM and non-REM sleep are as different from each other as
sleep is to waking. It is likely that the entire brain participates

in the sleep-wake cycles through all its neurotransmitters.

Sleep can be procured in a number of ways: by increasing 5-HT brain levels, by stimulating GABA, by suppressing NE and glutamate, or by antihistamine effects upon the H_1 receptor. Reduced firing by opening Cl^- channels or other methods of preventing depolarization will induce and sustain sleep. Decreased Ca^{++} should encourage sleep by reducing most neurotransmission.

Malignant carcinoids are tumors of the enterochromaffin cells of the intestine and contain enormous amounts of 5-HT. Carcinoids produce diarrhea and abdominal cramping. They have few mental effects because 5-HT passes through the blood-brain barrier with difficulty.

Apparently, a variety of biochemical bases for depression exist. Some may be due to catecholaminergic depletion, some to serotonergic depletion, or to combinations of the two. An increase in 5-HT receptors have been reported following electroconvulsive therapy. In one study depressed patients with low 5-hydroxyindoleacetic acid (5-HIAA) urine levels were ten times as likely to commit suicide as those with high 5-HIAA levels.

Histamine (H)

Histamine has many peripheral actions, bronchoconstriction, capillary vasodilation, enhanced capillary permeability, hypotension, and increased gastric secretion being a few. Whether histamine is a CNS transmitter is not yet fully established, but it is capable of producing behavioral responses when introduced intraventricularly. Histaminergic neurons have not yet been definitely identified.

The central action of histamine must include decreased arousal, thus accounting for the sedative effects of some H_1 antihistamines. In addition, histamine seems to play a role in food and water intake and the release of certain hormones.

Histamine has two subtype receptors. Stimulation of H_1 subtype receptors in the inner ear will reduce motion sickness. Antihistamines like dimenhydrinate (Dramamine) that act on H_1 receptors will relieve it. H_2 receptors increase gastric secretion and motility. Selective H_2 antagonists like cimetidine (Tagamet) will reduce acid secretion and are used in peptic ulcer therapy.

Amino Acids

Glutamate (Glutamic Acid) and Aspartate

These amino acids are general excitants of most neurons. Glutamate is widely distributed in the CNS, especially in the interneurons, and it increases ion conductance. Therefore it acts as a rapid depolarizer and intensifies firing rates.

Gamma Aminobutyric Acid (GABA) and Glycine

These are major inhibitors of most interneuronal transmissions. Both amino acids increase chloride conductance; therefore, they hyperpolarize the neuron and stop transmission. Picrotoxin is an antagonist of GABA, and strychnine antagonizes glycine. GABA-ergic neurons account for 30% of all neurotransmission in the CNS.

GABA is the restrainer of brain activity when behavioral sequences become unnecessary or redundant. Arousal, aggression, anxiety and excitation are reduced along with other hypervigilant behaviors.

Benzodiazepines apparently exert their effect by potentiating the GABA inhibitory response. The benzodiazepine receptor is situated in close proximity to the GABA receptor.

GABA raises the convulsive threshold, and the anticonvulsant effect of the benzodiazepines is probably mediated by this mechanism. Picrotoxin and bicuculine, since they are GABA antagonists, are convulsants.

Isoniazid (isonicotinic acid hydrazide, INH), an antitubercular agent, also causes convulsions. It acts to neutralize the effect of vitamin B_6 (pyridoxine), which is a coenzyme in the conversion of glutamic acid to GABA by glutamic acid decarboxylase (GAD). As a result, glutamic acid builds up in the neurons, GABA is decreased, and excitatory activity is intensified, provoking seizures. The breakdown of GABA to succinic aldehyde is mediated by GABA transminase.

Although other neurotransmitters have a dominant role in Parkinsonism—DA and ACh, for example—GABA also seems to contribute to that movement disorder. GABA levels are decreased in the EPS, and the number of GABA receptors in the substantia nigra is reduced. It could be that this event is secondary to the nigral degeneration of dopaminergic neurons. In Huntington's disease, a reduction of glutamic acid decarboxylase (GAD) activity in the basal ganglia is reported.

In epilepsy it has been found that a decreased GAD activity at the epileptic focus with reductions in GABA receptors and GABA spinal fluid content occur. Since the inhibitory action of GABA would be diminished, it is reasonable to assume that seizure thresholds would be lowered.

Anxiety states and insomnia have traditionally been treated with barbiturates. This class of drugs influences GABA transmission by interacting with the cell membrane close to the chloride channel, keeping it open for a longer time. This prolongs the GABA effect, increasing the inhibition of neurotransmission and producing sedation.

The benzodiazepines, on the other hand, attach to specific receptors in the vicinity of the GABA receptor, increasing its inhibitory action. An endogenous ligand for the benzodiazepine receptor has not been identified with certainty, although an anxiety-inducing peptide is suspected. It may be appropriate for an organism to possess an anxiety or fear-evoking neurotransmitter. Vigilance and arousal would be heightened, and the organism could prepare to focus on the external threat.

The ability of various benzodiazepines to bind to the benzodiazepine receptor parallels their therapeutic potency. The highest concentration of these receptors is to be found in the limbic system, the hippocampus and the olfactory bulb, thus accounting for their antianxiety effects. Their hypnosedative property might be attributable to receptor density in the limbic system.

Anxiety might be conceptualized as excessive firing in specific brain areas, like the limbic system. The hyperexcitability feeds back to GABA neurons, after which GABA is released, opening the chloride channels and inhibiting neuronal firing. The presence of benzodiazepines enhances GABA binding and intensifies the antianxiety effect. Sudden withdrawal of the benzodiazepine after prolonged use may induce a rebound hyperexcitability with symptoms of sedative withdrawal. Eventually, GABA homeostasis is restored. Rather than a withdrawal syndrome, discontinuance of the benzodiazepine may permit the reemergence of preexisting anxiety that had been suppressed by the drug.

Neuropeptides

A breakthrough in brain chemistry occurred during the 1970s when it was found that opioid peptides, relatively short chains of amino acids, were neurotransmitters at highly specific, saturable binding sites. Since then, enormous research efforts have been undertaken around the world to explore the variety and extent of neuropeptide transmission. Much of the effort has been directed at the endogenous opioid peptides. These are the internally produced peptides that are related pharmacologically to morphine. Their chemical structures are very different, but when examined in a three-dimensional configuration with consideration given to their electrical conformation, they come to resemble each other. A number of nonopioid peptides are known, and they will be discussed later.

Endogenous Opioid Peptides (Endorphins)

Although the term "endorphin" has been given to one of three classes of endogenous opioids, it will be used here to designate the entire group of internal peptides that have morphine-like characteristics. They consist of at least a dozen peptides produced in the brain and pituitary gland. The simplest and first identified were two 5-amino acid linkages, both of which contained the 4-amino acid sequence: tyrosine-glycine-glycine-phenylalanine. The fifth amino acid was either methionine or leucine. The met-enkephalin and leu-enkephalin sequences can also be found within other opioid peptides.

Beta endorphin is a 31-amino acid chain formed in the pituitary from a precursor, beta lipotropin. Actually, beta lipotropin itself is a split-off product of a protein called proopiomelanocortin (which originates in mRNA). It cleaves enzymatically into beta lipotropin, ACTH, and melano-stimulating hormone (MSH). It is appropriate that ACTH, which is released in response to stress or pain, be accompanied by beta endorphin, an analgesic. The role of MSH is less obvious. The dynorphins are potent peptides derived from prodynorphin. They contain 14 to 17 amino acids.

When synthetic endogenous or exogenous opioids are administered in a form that reaches the brain, both are antagonized by the same compounds, for example, naloxone (Narcan) and naltrexone (Trexan). Morphine-like withdrawal

TABLE II

THE OPIOID RECEPTORS

NAME	LIGANDS (EXAMPLES)	EFFECTS (EXAMPLES)
μ (mu)	Morphine and other opiates Beta endorphin Buprenorphine Pentazocine (antagonist) Naloxone (antagonist)	Analgesia Euphoria Respiratory depression Miosis Physical dependence
δ (delta)	Enkephalins Beta endorphin Butorphanol (Stadol)	Euphoria Analgesia
κ (kappa)	Morphine Naloxone Dynorphins Nalbuphine Pentazocine Bupremorphine Butorphanol	Analgesia Sedation Miosis Psychotomimetic (?)
σ (sigma)	Pentazocine Nalbuphine Phencyclidine	Dysphoria Psychotomimetic
ε (epsilon)	Beta endorphin	?
Cough suppressant	Dextromethorphan (naloxone has no affinity)	Antitussive
λ (lambda)	?	?

symptoms are observed when synthetic endogenous opioids are given and suddenly stopped, or if a narcotic antagonist is given in the course of their administration. If an animal has been made tolerant to the endorphins, the opiates will sustain the tolerance. These phenomena and others indicate that both the internal opioids and the external narcotics act similarly, and both have an affinity for similar opioid receptors. In fact, small amounts of morphine itself have apparently been identified in some laboratory animals not given morphine or similar opioids.

Opiopeptides are capable of functioning as neurotransmitters, neuromodulators or neurohormones. When they act as transmitters, the peptides evoke a slower, but more sustained response than the biogenic amines. As modulators they have a variable, nonspecific impact on neuronal sensitivity. As blood-borne hormones, they affect many brain functions and slow gastrointestinal transit time.

The opioid peptides modulate the sensation of pain by altering the emotional implications of the painful experience, in other words, the suffering. In addition, the transmission within pain-carrying neurons is attenuated. Opioids are involved at the reward centers, in feeding behavior, growth, sensitivity to hemorrhagic shock, and in the consolidation of memory. Overall, the opioid peptides counteract the impact of physical and psychological stress and tend to reestablish the organism's homeostasis.

Opioids and opioid antagonists have recognition sites on the neurons that they influence, shaped and electrically charged to receive them, rather like a credit card is recognized and received by a banking machine.

At least five opioid receptors have been postulated and more will be identified, each with varying affinities for the opioid agonists and antagonists. They are called mu (for morphine), delta, kappa (for ketocyclazocine), sigma (also a PCP receptor) and epsilon.

Originally, interest in endorphin receptors was focused on their analgesic activity and their possible relationship to opioid addiction. Currently, these interests remain, but work has been expanded to many other areas. It is now evident that opioid recognition sites are found in centers involved in emotionality, neurohormone secretion and cognition, well beyond matters of pain and opioid dependence.

The Opioid Agonists

Representative of the agonists are derivatives of opium, like morphine, heroin, codeine, hydromorphone (Dilaudid), hydrocodone (Hycodan), oxymorphone (Numorphan) and oxycodone (Percodan). These are mu receptor agonists, and some also have affinity for the kappa receptor. In addition, a number of synthetic compounds that resemble morphine in their activity are used therapeutically, including meperidine (Demerol), methadone (Dolophine), fentanyl (Sublimaze) and propoxyphene (Darvon).

The rewarding effects of a drug like morphine are mediated by dopaminergic neurons over the ventral tegmentum and onto the nucleus accumbens. When morphine is injected directly into the ventral tegmentum of rats, physical dependence does not occur. Injections into the perventricular gray, an area involved in pain transmission, does produce physical dependence. Thus, it appears that the analgesic effects of opioids can be separated from their dependency-producing effects.

The euphoric effects of the major stimulants also are involved in increased firing of the dopamine system; therefore, injecting a combination of heroin and cocaine (speedball) makes pharmacologic sense but not physiologic sense, since both drugs eventually depress the breathing center.

The endogenous agonists like the enkephalins, the dynorphins and the alpha and beta endorphin groups are representative of the known internal opioids. Analgesia produced by these compounds can be prolonged by inactivating the peptidases responsible for their breakdown.

From our knowledge of the endorphin system, it may be possible to redefine insensitivity to pain, or stoicism, the ability to endure pain. While stoic attitudes can be trained or learned by life experiences, some resilience to feeling pain may be genetic. People with naturally elevated endorphins, or those with more than average numbers of opioid receptors, may have a congenital elevation of pain thresholds.

A poor tolerance to pain, on the other hand, could be related to congenitally low endorphin levels or a paucity of receptors. A genetically determined high concentration or release of Substance P would also produce low pain thresholds. The response to pain is, in part, a learned or conditioned response and is amenable to early life modification from family or cultural attitudes to pain. The meaning of pain is an important variable. Studies have shown that war wounds ordinarily require less analgesia than identical wounds experienced in civilian accidents. In the first instance the wound may signify a trip home from the battlefield; in the second instance it may represent negative implications such as the loss of a job, hospital expenses, or a lawsuit.

Reports of placebos increasing endorphin production would explain why a third of the population obtains relief from nonactive drugs. Additional studies are needed to confirm this point. Likewise, investigations reporting increased endorphin availability during long-distance running, acupuncture, and hypnosis require replication.

Because of the discovery of internal pain modulators that act on the same receptor sites as external opioids, consideration must be given concerning our cultural attitudes toward relief of pain and suffering. Pain relief afforded by the endogenous opioids is rarely complete. This would indicate that retention of the pain signal is congruent with survival and should not be obliterated lest the painful process require remediation. When opiates are provided, an optimal effect would be that the patient is no longer suffering, but that a decreased awareness of the pain remains.

The new knowledge about internal opioids and about their specific receptors that provide relief of pain and dysphoria could require a reconsideration of our social attitudes toward opium derivatives and synthetic narcotics. It might be argued that since naturally occurring substances for the relief of noxious states are present, why should a societal taboo against drugs that mimic their action exist? Shouldn't these drugs be as readily available as food supplements for those who wish to reduce their suffering?

From what is known of our endogenous mechanisms for assuaging psychological and physical distress, ready, uncontrolled access to opiates cannot be recommended. The endorphins provide partial relief so that remedial action can be taken against the source of the distress. Under normal conditions, physical dependence on the endorphins probably does not occur. However, physical dependence is seen when users have ample access to opiates. It is unlikely that we are wise enough to use the narcotics as discriminatingly as the brain uses the endogenous opioids. The disasters of overuse by unsupervised individuals are never seen when the internal analgesic mechanisms are functioning.

When exogenous opioids are administered, they produce a deficiency of endorphins which is restored only over time. Thus, the discovery of the endorphin system hardly seems to be an excuse to provide opiates to those who want them for whatever purposes. We also have a phencyclidine (PCP) receptor. Should this permit the indiscriminate use of phencyclidine? What is not perceived is that brain regulatory mechanisms prevent excessive reward center stimulation by downregulation. Brain circuitry permits momentary ecstasy or prolonged pleasure. Apparently, sustained ecstasy is neuro-physiologically impossible.

Opioid Antagonists

Naloxone (Narcan) and naltrexone (Trexan) are pure antagonists. They compete with mu, kappa and delta agonists at the receptor sites and displace them if they are already attached. If naloxone is administered before a painful stimulus, the organism becomes more sensitive to pain because endogenous opioids are unable to bind to the receptor.

Aversive emotions induce endorphin production. Fear, panic, phobias and stress increase endorphin levels. The presence of opioid receptors in the limbic system indicate that endorphins function to relieve dysphoria and modulate the organism's response to emotional trauma.

Endogenous antagonists have been identified. Their function in the living organism is under study. One of them, β-endorphin-1-27, is believed to be five times more potent than naloxone. Another antagonist is a peptide also found in the intestine and gall bladder—cholecystokinin (CCK). A close interaction between CCK and the opioid peptides exists. Morphine is known to deplete brain CCK. When CCK is administered to animals, it acts like an opioid antagonist. It may be that CCK plays some role in tolerance and withdrawal from opioids.

When acting as a hormone, CCK stimulates gall bladder contraction, opening the common duct sphincter, and increasing intestinal motility. Opioids will oppose these actions, contracting the common duct sphincter and decreasing gut motility. These effects of opioids give rise to the complaints of constipation by heroin addicts and patients being treated with other opiates. It is also the basis of the antidiarrheal effects of diphenoxylate (Lomotil), a weak opioid.

Agonist-Antagonists

Some drugs have varying degrees of both agonistic and antagonistic activity. Nalorphine (Nalline), for example, is a mu antagonist, a partial kappa agonist and a sigma agonist. Pentazocine (Talwin) is a mu antagonist and a kappa and sigma agonist. At average doses pentazocine induces analgesia and some respiratory depression; at high doses dysphoria and psychotomimetic effects are seen. In heroin addicts withdrawal can be precipitated by pentazocine. It has been used for its euphoric effects in combination with pyribenzamine as Ts (Talwin) and blues (pyribenzamine). The antihistamine pyribenzamine potentiates mu agonist activity, thereby making the pentazocine more euphorogenic.

The antagonistic effects of pentazocine are so weak that naloxone had to be added to its formulation in order to increase its aversive effect when used parenterally by opioid-dependent people. Nalbuphine (Nubain) resembles pentazocine as a mu antagonist, a partial agonist at the kappa receptor and a sigma agonist. As with pentazocine, nalbuphine in high doses will produce withdrawal effects.

Buprenorphine (marketed as Temgesic in England and Germany and Buprenex in the United States) is a partial mu agonist. In opioid-dependent individuals who have recently become abstinent, buprenorphine will suppress early withdrawal signs. On the other hand, in actively using opioid-dependent people buprenorphine will precipitate withdrawal. This suggests some antagonistic effects. Instances of buprenorphine dependence have been reported in countries where it is approved for prescription use.

Other Neuropeptide Transmitters

A variety of other transmitter peptides, whose numbers will surely increase, are found in the CNS. Many of them also serve as hormones. Neuropeptides are derived from prohormones by a splitting of segments of the molecule by a peptidase. The prohormones are sections of mRNA.

Substance P

Substance P seems to be a transmitter of pain-related information in the dorsal horn of the spinal cord and in the brain. It is found in the slow pain fibers, those that transmit at a rate of 0.5 to 2 meters per second. Endorphins are located in the same areas as Substance P and inhibit its release. In the periaqueductal gray of the thalamus a similar antagonism to Substance P exists. Electrical stimulation of this area stimulates endorphin activity and relieves pain. This technique is useful in treatment of some types of otherwise intractable pain.

Vasopressin (Antidiuretic Hormone, ADH)

This antidiuretic hormone and vasoconstrictor is also a neurotransmitter in the hypothalamus. It participates in the release of ACTH. ADH helps regulate body temperature, fluid balance and visceral activity. It seems to be a factor in the coagulation process. Alcohol inhibits the secretion of ADH and in that way alcohol acts as a diuretic. Diabetes insipidus is often due to a failure of ADH secretion from the posterior pituitary. Vasopressin agonists improve memory performance.

Angiotensin II

Angiotensin II, a neuropeptide, is a potent initiator of fluid intake. Thus both vasopressin, by conserving fluid, and angiotensin II, by increasing fluid consumption, act to cope with blood loss and dehydration. Angiotensin II promotes the secretion of vasopressin in fluid-depleted animals. Our response to dehydration is orchestrated by these two neuropeptides, which results in behaviors that seek relief from the feeling of thirst, namely, the drinking of fluids and the conservation of blood volume. When angiotensin production is reduced by preventing its polypeptide precursors from splitting off the angiotensin II molecule, hypertension improves, possibly by reducing body fluid volume.

Oxytocin

Another transmitter-hormone secreted in the posterior pituitary is oxytocin. After release into the bloodstream it stimulates uterine contractions especially during labor, stimulates the ejection of milk, and assists in the regulation of blood pressure. It also plays a role in regulating food intake. Both oxytocin and vasopressin have a role to play in learning, memory and improved behavioral performance.

Additional Neuropeptides

Somatostatin

The somatostatins are capable of inhibiting the release of many hormones like growth hormone, insulin, thyrotropin, parathyroid hormones, and a number of gastrointestinal hormones. It is not to be confused with growth hormone-releasing factor which stimulates release of growth hormone from the anterior pituitary gland. In general, it is a depressant of CNS activity.

Neurotensin

Neurotensin is a very potent hypothermic agent. Its analgesic activity is further evidence that nonopioid analgesia occurs in the CNS. Enhanced release of adrenocorticotrophic hormone (ACTH), follicle-stimulating hormone (FSH), and lutein-stimulating hormone (LH) indicates that neurotensin acts as a releasing hormone. It is also claimed to enhance memory.

In addition, insulin, glucagon, bombesin, and secretin are neurohormones. They are also to be found in the gastrointestinal tract. Bradykinin, carnosine and calcitonin are peptides that also seem to have a function in the brain. These and other chemicals like the prostaglandins appear to modulate the level of excitation of certain neurons. Cholecystokinin is often to be found in dopaminergic neurons, and VIP (vasoactive intestinal peptide) colocates with ACh.

Neurohormones

Information within the CNS is transmitted primarily along neurons by electrochemical means to the synaptic gap, where the information bit becomes a purely chemical transaction, apparently for purposes of modulating the signal. Another information delivery system involves not only the brain, but also other organs, especially the endocrine glands. This system is controlled in the hypothalamus, a sort of master control area at the base of the brain. Many of the neurotransmitters from the cerebral cortex and limbic system bring data to the hypothalamus for integration and action. It is here that releasing hormones provide orders to the pituitary gland to secrete hormones that will activate the thyroid, adrenal cortex, gonads, pineal gland, and other structures outside the brain. In addition, inhibitory hormones are produced—hormones that will stop the releasing hormone's activity. Another hypothalamic function is the regulation of the heart, gut and other peripheral structures via the autonomic nervous system. Along with brainstem structures, the hypothalamus delivers parasympathetic (acetylcholine) and sympathetic (norepineph-rine and epinephrine) transmissions to the viscera, blood ves-sels, muscles, and skin for coordinated regulatory control.

Some of the hypothalamic releasing and inhibiting hor-mones are delivered to special cells in the posterior pituitary. In fact, this area is an extension of the hypothalamus and consists of neural tissue. The posterior pituitary hormones oxytocin and angiotensin have already been mentioned. As can be seen from Table IV, the posterior pituitary secretes vasopressin. In addition to their effects upon the blood vessels, kidney, and uterus, these hormones serve as neurotransmitters.

The anterior pituitary hormones regulate the secretion of the thyroid, adrenal cortex, and gonads. In addition, prolactin controls breast development and milk secretion, and growth hormone increases protein synthesis. (See Table III.)

Some of the hypothalamic-pituitary hormones also serve as neurotransmitters within the neuron, modifying the action of a primary transmitter. Other hormones made in organs dis-tant from the brain have been found to serve as transmitters or modulators of the neural signal. Cholecystokinin (CCK), bombesin, testosterone, and estrogen are only a few of the substances known to influence neuronal function. Estrogen and testosterone receptors in the hypothalmus, for example, differentiate brain activity and structure to the point that male and female brains can be distinguished macroscopically. In certain hypothalamic areas differences in size can be seen without a microscope. CCK may be the food satiety factor; and bombesin appears to induce eating behavior and be involved in sensory processing. Both are synthesized in the intestine.

A prime characteristic of the hormones made in the hypothalamus and pituitary gland is close control of their man-ufacture by feedback mechanisms from their target hormones, by the influence of other hormones, and by information from the brain. An example of how corticosteroid levels are con-

TABLE III

HYPOTHALAMIC REGULATORY HORMONES

The following hormones control the release or inhibition of pituitary hormones.

HORMONE	ABBREVIATION	THERAPEUTIC USE
1. Corticotropin releasing factor	CRF	Diagnosis of adrenal-cortical insuffiency
2. Thyrotropin releasing hormone	TRH	Diagnosis of primary vs secondary hypothyroidism
3. Leutinizing hormone-releasing hormone	LH-RH	Treat cryptorchism (undescended testicles), induce puberty and ovulation. Treat precocious puberty
4. Follicle stimulating hormone-releasing hormone	FSH-RH	—
5. Growth hormone-releasing factor	GH-RF	—
6. Growth hormone release-inhibiting hormone (somatostatin)	GH-RIH	Suppresses release of many endocrine hormones
7. Prolactin releasing factor (dopamine?)	PRF	—
8. Prolactin release-inhibiting hormone	PR-IH	
9. Melanocyte stimulating hormone-releasing factor	MRF	—
10. Melanocyte stimulating hormone release-inhibiting factor	MIF	—

TABLE IV

PITUITARY HORMONES

I. ANTERIOR PITUITARY	ABBREVIATION	THERAPEUTIC USE
1. Follicle stimulating hormone	FSH	Infertility, cryptorchism
2. Leutinizing hormone	LH	Infertility, cryptorchism
3. Thyrotropin (thyroid stimulating hormone)	TSH	Diagnosis of thyroid disorders
4. Adrenocorticotrophic hormone	ACTH	Regulates salt, sugar, electrolytes, antiflammatory, etc.
5. Growth hormone	GH	Hypopituitary dwarfism
6. Prolactin	—	—
7. Melanocyte stimulating hormone	MSH	—

II. POSTERIOR PITUITARY		
1. Vasopressin	ADH, VP	Antidiuretic, diabetes insipidus
2. Oxytocin	—	Milk production and letdown, induction of labor

trolled is given below. Similar arrangements exist for other neurohormones.

1. Influences from neurotransmitters in the cortex and limbic system induce the secretion of corticotropin-releasing factor (CRF) in the hypothalamus.

2. Via the portal venous system between the hypothalamus and the pituitary, CRF occupies receptors in the anterior pituitary and stimulates the release of corticotropin (ACTH).

3. Via the systemic circulation ACTH arrives at the adrenal cortex and induces secretion of cortisol and other corticosteroids.

4. Cortisol acts at a number of target organs regulating water, electrolyte, protein, fat and glucose metabolism (stress response).

5. The levels of the corticosteroids in the blood feed back to ACTH- and CRF-producing cells to invoke a decrease or increase in the production of CRF or ACTH.

Mention should be made of two other hypothalamic regulatory hormones. Thyrotropin-releasing hormone (TRH) is a tripeptide. It contains three amino acids linked together. In addition to its function as a releaser of thyroid-stimulating hormone, it is active in many other parts of the brain. It increases spontaneous motor activity and enhances DA, NE and ACh actions. TRH reverses the effects of barbiturates, alcohol, diazepam and other sedatives. It may have a role to play in reducing the depressant effects of these drugs under overdose conditions.

Leutinizing hormone-releasing hormone (LH-RH) has been shown to activate mating behavior in vertebrates. This activity fits in well with its hormonal function—that of preparing the female genitalia for pregnancy.

Principles of Neurotransmission

Before a chemical can be considered a synaptic messenger or
ligand, it must demonstrate the following functions:

1. It should be capable of being synthesized
within the neuron or be delivered from other
neurons or glial cells.

2. It must attach to specific receptors on the
postsynaptic neuron.

3. It must be released from neuronal terminals
into the synapse usually by Ca^{++} dependent release.

4. When the transmitter is provided from
exogenous sources, it must mimic the effects of
the endogenous transmitter, providing it crosses
the blood-brain barrier.

5. Catabolizing enzymes must be present to inactivate the transmitter.

6. Exogenous antagonists must antagonize the
endogenous transmitter.

It is no longer necessary to postulate that every neuron
has a single specific transmitter, since current information indicates that more than one transmitter can be used by a neuron.
For example, dopamine and a neuropeptide may function together. Dopamine provides the chemical signal while the
neuropeptide modulates or prolongs the signal.

Depolarization increases transmission by increasing Na^+
or Ca^{++} influx. Hyperpolarization by increasing Cl^- or K^+
influx blocks transmission. Stimulation of an excitatory

neuron excites postsynaptic activity. Stimulating an inhibitory neuron induces inhibition. Inhibiting an inhibitory neuron causes stimulation by reduction of inhibitory activity. It appears that much of neuronal transmission is inhibitory in nature.

When excessive numbers of transmitter molecules are available to the receptor over time, a decrease in the receptor sites can be counted. This is called downregulation and may account for certain types of tolerance. At any rate the reduction of receptors will produce desensitization, a reduced neuronal reactivity. Such a situation might occur when heroin consistently occupies opioid binding sites. Downregulation occurs and tolerance is noted. The desensitized postsynaptic cell will not respond to average amounts of heroin, but increased amounts are required to obtain an opioid effect, which induces greater levels of tolerance.

The reverse situation occurs when decreased numbers of transmitter molecules are available at the postsynaptic receptor sites. This leads to upregulation with an increased number of sensitized receptors. Such a condition would occur during receptor blockade. An example is the use of neuroleptics, Thorazine, for instance, over a long period.

Thorazine blocks DA receptors, inducing upregulation. Additional dopamine receptors appear on the postsynaptic membrane. At this point the postsynaptic neuron is hypersensitive, and if the blockade is ended, even average amounts of dopamine can cause a movement disorder called tardive dyskinesia. The condition is treated by dopamine antagonists or by reestablishing the dopamine blockade.

The postsynaptic receptor contains specific recognition sites that are situated at the outer layer of the membrane. The remainder of the lipoprotein receptor molecule, the transducer, extends into the inner part of the membrane and relays the signal. The signal will regulate the opening or closing of the postsynaptic neuron's ion channels determining whether or not the neuron will fire. Other effects would include activation of second messengers (the presynaptic transmitter is the first messenger), which determine whether synaptic transmission will occur or whether neuronal proteins will be made.

A second messenger system exists within the postsynaptic cell. It is slower but lasts longer than first messenger signals. Both messenger systems activate the enzyme adenylate cyclase to produce cAMP (cyclic adenosine monophosphate). It can alter membrane conductance, activate enzymes, or change the rate of protein synthesis.

The effectiveness of neurotransmission depends upon a number of variables. Factors that influence transmission would include:

1. Changes in amount of the precursor available.

2. Changes in the enzyme level that transforms the precursor into the transmitter.

3. Alterations in the amount of and exposure to the metabolizing enzymes that degrade the transmitter into its inactive end product.

4. Variations in the rate of discharge of vesicular contents into the synapse.

5. Blockage of the reuptake of the excess transmitter from the synapse back into the vesicles. Neuropeptide transmitters have no reuptake system.

6. The degree of Ca^{++} flux into the neuron. The greater the Ca^{++} flux, the more prolonged is the transmitter discharge.

7. The density and sensitivity of the postsynaptic receptors.

8. Interference with the second messenger system.

Drugs act upon one or more of the above variables:

1. A precursor like the amino acid tryptophan may increase the amount of serotonin available.

2. A drug can block the enzyme which changes the precursor into the transmitter. Alphamethyl-tyrosine (not available as a medicine) blocks the enzyme tyrosine hydroxylase that converts the amino acid tyrosine to dopa. Since it is the rate-limiting enzyme for subsequent production of all catecholamines, it therefore decreases the amount of dopamine, norepinephrine, and epinephrine produced.

3. The drug may act to block the metabolizing enzyme. Monoamine oxidase inhibitors (MAOIs) will inactivate the amine oxidases, preventing the degradation of biogenic amines like serotonin, dopamine, and norepinephrine. For example, MAOIs make norepinephrine more available at the receptors and can improve depressive states.

4. The drug may displace the natural ligand or its agonists at the receptor. For example, naloxone (Narcan) will displace endorphins or heroin at opioid binding sites antagonizing their effects. Atropine acts in a similar fashion at muscarinic receptors, and curare at nicotinic receptors. Propranolol (Inderal) is an antagonist to norepinephrine at beta adrenergic receptors.

5. The drug may mimic the action of the ligand or will increase receptor activity. Clonidine activates $alpha_2$ adrenergic receptors and thus reduces the autonomic symptoms of the opioid

withdrawal syndrome. Apomorphine and bromocriptine activate the dopamine receptor.

6. The drug may alter the receptor protein interfering with receptor activity. Cytotoxic agents change receptor protein configurations.

7. The drug may block access to the receptor. The antipsychotic drugs block the access of dopamine to its receptors in the limbic system, producing their antipsychotic actions, and in the basal ganglia, inducing their extrapyramidal effects.

8. The drug may block reuptake of excess transmitter from the synapse. In so doing it increases its availability at the postsynaptic receptors. Cocaine, amphetamines and tricyclic antidepressants interfere with the reuptake of monoamines like dopamine, norepinephrine, and serotonin. With the increased access of these monoamines, euphoriant or antidepressant effects are noted.

9. The drug may block the entry of the transmit ter into the storage vesicles and permit it to be metabolized in the cytoplasm. Reserpine (Serpasil) prevents the entry of norepinephrine into the protective vesicle, exposing it to MAO and depleting norepinephrine. Reserpine occasionally causes depression.

10. The substance may act as a false transmitter, occupying the receptor but not transmitting the signal. Octopamine can occupy some norepinephrine receptors.

3

The Chemistry of Addiction

Slowly, the biochemical substrate of becoming and remaining drug dependent is becoming clearer. When patients are asked why they became involved, then overinvolved, with some drug, the response is some variation of "to feel better," or that they hoped to obtain relief from psychological or physical distress.

"To feel better" means many things. It is the rescue from boredom, surcease from the meaninglessness of existence, relief from the inability to enjoy the pleasures of existence or to cope with real or imagined stresses of everyday life. Some people appear to suffer more than most. They spend a good part of their lifetimes struggling to evade distress, unpleasure, and other noxious feelings.

It might be assumed that some people are dysphoric (unhappy) or anhedonic (unable to feel pleasure) because of the learned behavior and mental attitudes of their earlier years. It may be that their view of life through somber glasses is the result of interminable misfortunes. Perhaps there is a not yet uncovered biological basis for constant misery, or what may be even worse, for not being able to feel anything deeply at all.

It is easy to postulate that the reinforcement centers in the ventral tegmentum, the locus ceruleus, the mediolateral frontal cortex, or the nucleus accumbens have an inborn deficiency of catecholamines or that the receptors are hyposensitive. Alternatively, perhaps the endogenous opioids are congenitally in short supply or the delta opioid receptor is deficient in quantity or quality. Will diagnoses like "hypoendorphism" or "opioid receptor insufficiency" or "hypodopaminosis" ever be made with reliability? The early work in this area indicates that the possibility exists.

To glance at another aspect of mood disorders, it would make some kind of sense to say that for each troubled person there would be a preferred drug of dependence. For the depressed person, some stimulant potion might be preferred. A chronic worrier might select an antianxiety agent. For those in pain, an analgesic might be chosen. From clinical experience this reasonable assumption does not hold. We find some depressed persons consuming depressants; and often enough, manics seek out stimulants. The schizophrenic with a certain difficulty in keeping in touch with reality may prefer hallucinogens. Besides, what can be said of our polydrug abusers who employ every available mood-altering substance—uppers, downers, inners, and outers? It seems that what is available at the moment determines what is used, rather than specific mood modulators being selected for specific ailments.

What follows is an attempt to explain the mode of action of pleasure-giving and pain-relieving agents that are abused. This will not be easy because we are neither so ignorant that a few words will suffice, nor so knowledgeable that the neurochemistry of addiction is at hand, with some master data bank printing out the answers.

But first we should try to understand the chemical basis of general concepts like dependence, tolerance, withdrawal, and other phenomena associated with the addicted condition.

Drug Dependence

It is not helpful to separate psychological dependence (habituation) from physical dependence (addiction). The psychological need to continue using is a part of addiction along with the added burden of the requirement to avoid the physical withdrawal sickness. Some drugs, such as cannabis, have minor withdrawal effects. Yet people still have considerable difficulty ridding themselves of the habit. Other drugs, like cocaine, are so compelling (reinforcing) that whatever physical dependence exists is overshadowed by the craving to compulsively continue to use the drug. So a definition of dependence should include loss of control over usage and continued involvement with the drug despite serious adverse consequences. Drug dependence also includes physiologic elements—tolerance development and the emergence of withdrawal effects following discontinuance.

Tolerance

The psychophysiology of tolerance has variable causes. One is that the liver and other organs learn how to deal with the repeated use of the drug, either by metabolizing it more effectively by enzyme induction or by excreting it more efficiently (dispositional tolerance). Tolerance also develops because the target cells begin to adapt better to the presence of the drug, perhaps by downregulation (pharmacodynamic tolerance). Receptor affinity, activity of ion movements, enzymes regulating Ca^{++} or cAMP, or other changes of sensitivity within the neuron are further possibilities. Another is the organism's capacity to learn to adjust to the effects of the drug by behavioral adaptation (behavioral tolerance).

Tachyphylaxis

Tachyphylaxis is an accelerated development of tolerance. Only one or a few doses of the drug will produce a significant decrease or complete loss of reactivity to the drug. LSD provides a prime example of tachyphylaxis. It is without effect after three days of regular usage. Recovery of sensitivity occurs within a few days. The psychostimulants tend to show rapid tolerance when large amounts are used for short periods.

Tachyphylaxis may represent the rapid exhaustion of a neurotransmitter or an accelerated loss of receptor sensitivity.

Kindling

Kindling can be thought of as the opposite of tolerance development. It is analogous to igniting a wood fire. It spreads very slowly at first, hardly seeming to progress, then suddenly a brisk blaze burns. If a drug is capable of producing some symptom, regular use of the drug at the original dosage level may evoke the symptom, not after the first dose, but after multiple doses. In animals, repeated average doses of cocaine have induced generalized convulsions over time. Human grand mal convulsions in connection with cocaine use may also be due to kindling, but that possibility has not been tested in a research setting. The basis for kindling can be a sensitization of the receptors, enhanced production of the neurotransmitter involved, or channeling, since the regular use of a neural pathway facilitates subsequent transmission.

Cross Tolerance and Cross Dependence

After tolerance develops to one drug, the individual will also manifest tolerance to other drugs in the same class and may show tolerance to drugs of related classes. Thus alcohol induces a degree of tolerance to the sedative-hypnotics.

Cross dependence exists when a person is dependent on one drug, and other drugs in that class or in closely related classes will prevent withdrawal effects. Methadone maintenance is an instance of cross dependence, with methadone taking over the dependence on heroin. Drugs that demonstrate cross tolerance will also show cross dependence to each other. The phenomena of cross tolerance and cross dependence are believed to be the use of similar neural conduction mechanisms by similarly acting drugs.

The Withdrawal Syndrome

The hallmark of the withdrawal syndrome is rebound hyper- or hypoexcitability. When a person dependent on CNS depressants suddenly stops using, or when a narcotic antagonist is administered to opiate addicts, a clinical picture opposite to that produced by the CNS depressant emerges. Instead of sedation, restlessness, autonomic hyperactivity and agitation come forth. If sufficient amounts of a stimulant have been taken over weeks or months, the abstinence syndrome produces a picture of psychic depression and hypersomnia. It would seem as though the adaptive maneuvers of the body to the abused drug had suppressed the CNS and its autonomic manifestations. Rebound symptoms will emerge when brain levels of the stimulant or depressant are lowered.

In the instance of opioids, benzodiazepines and certain other drugs, brain levels may be high; but if an antagonist is present, it will displace the drugs from their stereospecific binding sites and evoke withdrawal. Therefore, the preempting of sufficient receptor sites can provoke withdrawal effects that last until the endogenous transmitter, which had been suppressed, is restored.

It has been shown that opioids suppress NE locus ceruleus (arousal) activity. This suppression can be reversed by naloxone or naltrexone. Many of the autonomic and mood disturbances encountered in opioid withdrawal can be reversed by clonidine, an alpha$_1$ adrenergic agonist. The reinforcing activity of opioids occur at the level of their specific opioid receptors.

The time required to produce physical dependence varies with the drug involved. However, the relevant neurons must have been exposed to sufficient concentrations of the drug over days to months to produce an abstinence syndrome. It was for this reason that earlier textbooks on pharmacology stated that physical dependence on cocaine did not occur. Cocaine is a short-acting drug and must be taken frequently, as it is now, to manifest withdrawal phenomena.

Protracted Abstinence Syndrome

After recovery from the acute withdrawal effects, an opioid-dependent person may experience prolonged residual signs and symptoms indicative of continuing psychophysiological changes. EEG alterations, an abnormal response to an opiate injection, difficulty in dealing with stress or pain, and mild deviations of vital signs may be present for months. It is believed that these protracted symptoms may make such a person more vulnerable to relapse.

Mode of Action

Stimulants

Cocaine

The most abused stimulants include cocaine, amphetamine, methylphenidate (Ritalin) and phenmetrazine (Preludin). Cocaine is the most reinforcing chemical known. When access to cocaine is unlimited, animals will continue to press a bar for a cocaine reward until they are exhausted or convulsing. Other ordinarily pleasurable activities, such as food and sex, will be ignored in preference to cocaine. The effects of amphetamine are difficult to distinguish from cocaine's except for the longer action of amphetamine.

While tolerance will develop over time to certain effects

TABLE V

COCAINE: SYMPTOMS, TOXICITY & TRANSMITTERS

SYMPTOMS	COMPLICATIONS	NEUROTRANSMITTERS
Paranoid thinking mode	Paranoid psychosis	DA ↑
Hyperthermia	Heat stroke	NE ↑
Hypertension	Cerebral hemorrhage	NE ↑
Convulsions	Status epilepticus	NE ↑, GABA ↓
Tachycardia	Ventricular arrythmias	NE ↑
Hyperpnea	Apnea	NE ↑
Dilated pupils	—	NE ↑
Anorexia	Malnutrition	NE ↑
Insomnia	—	NE ↑

PROLONGED USE

Euphoria	Dysphoria, depression	DA ↑, later DA ↓
Hypersexuality	Hyposexuality	DA ↑, later DA ↓

of these drugs (euphoria, hyperthermia, anorexia, etc.), other effects such as convulsions, paranoia, and cardiac and pulmonary effects may kindle.

It is believed that the rewarding effects of cocaine are secondary to the availability of large numbers of dopamine molecules at the postsynaptic receptors in the brain centers that evoke pleasure and elation. These sensations result primarily from cocaine's ability to prevent the reuptake of DA back into the presynaptic neuron, thereby presenting the DA receptor sites with more DA over a longer interval. The free DA in the synapse is metabolized by the enzyme COMT and cannot be reused. Following a cocaine "run," DA is reduced or exhausted, accounting for the dysphoric mood (the "coke blues") and for the inability to enjoy ordinarily pleasurable events. When DA stores are replenished, the ability to enjoy returns. In addition to the blockade of the reentry of DA back into the presynaptic vesicles, there is evidence that DA is also released in larger amounts by cocaine.

Other monoamines, particularly NE and 5-HT, are similarly affected by cocaine, producing psychophysiologic effects mentioned in Table V.

Amphetamine

Chronic high-dose amphetamine and methamphetamine exposure is neurotoxic, producing dopaminergic nerve terminal degeneration and a marked decrease in receptor sites. This is particularly noted in the striatum. It is due to the oxidation of some of the dopamine to 6-hydroxydopamine, a specific DA toxin. Intravenous amphetamine abuse has receded, but oral abuse of the amphetamine group remains significant. The mechanism of action of the amphetamines mimics that of cocaine and includes the following:

1. An inhibitor of monoamine reuptake.

2. A catecholamine agonist.

3. A releaser of monoamines into the synapse.

4. An MAOI preventing catecholamine breakdown within the neuron.

All of these actions result in an initial increase of DA, NE and 5-HT at their receptor sites. Following extended high-dose use, depletion of the monoamines takes place so that a reversal of some of the earlier symptoms will occur (elation to depression, for example).

Other Anorexiants

Other anorexiant agents besides amphetamines are occasionally abused. However, their euphoriant action tends to be weaker than the compounds discussed above. In fact, mazindol (Sanorex), fenfluramine (Pondimin) and phenyl-propanolamine (Dexatrim, etc.) do not act as reinforcers in animals and are usually not euphoriant in humans. Methylphenidate (Ritalin) is a stimulant used for attention-deficit disorders. It has a significant abuse potential. Outbreaks of dependence on phenmetrazine (Preludin), a weight control medication, are known.

Caffeine

Caffeine is a relatively mild stimulant, but it does increase wakefulness and produce some increase in the flow of thought. Euphoria is rarely reported, and even when the dose is increased to above average amounts, an amphetamine-like effect cannot be achieved. Instead, anxiety, tremulousness, restlessness, and rare seizures will occur.

Caffeine has many effects upon the CNS. The most likely action that explains its stimulant property is that caffeine blocks adenosine receptors, thereby inhibiting the release of certain neurotransmitters. Since the action of most of these is inhibitory, a mild excitatory effect can result.

Hallucinogens

LSD Series (Mescaline, Psilocybin, etc.)

Since these compounds show similar clinical manifestations, exhibit cross tolerance to each other, and are affected by the same antagonists, they are believed to have similar mechanisms of action. LSD (lysergic acid diethylamide) and its analogues inhibit the release of 5-HT. LSD may act as a false transmitter by attaching itself to the 5-HT postsynaptic receptor sites and not permitting serotonergic activity. Nonhallucinogenic ergot alkaloids that have similar properties are known. We are far from understanding how the psychotomimetic drugs produce their profound changes in mental functioning.

One speculation about the manner by which hallucinogens manifest their impressive alterations of mood, perception and thought is that the pontine raphe, a major center of 5-HT activity, serves as a filtering station for incoming sensory stimuli. It screens the flood of sensations and percepts, eliminating those that are unimportant, irrelevant, or commonplace. A drug like LSD may disrupt the sorting process, allowing a surge of sensory data and an overload of brain circuits.

Dehabituation, in which the familiar becomes novel, is noted under LSD. It may also be caused by lowering the sensory gates by inhibition of raphe activity. LSD is a 4-substituted tryptamine. Other hallucinogenic tryptamines include DMT (dimethyltryptamine), bufotenine (5-hydroxy-DMT), psilocin (4-hydroxy-DMT) and psilocybin (4-phosphoryl-

DMT). Mescaline is a phenethylamine, but it demonstrates cross tolerance to the tryptamine hallucinogens. All of these agents inhibit raphe firing, as does 5-HT. These psychotomimetics also have an affinity for a subset of DA receptors. Their combined action on 5-HT and DA receptors could account for the well-known spectacular effects on mental function.

MDA, MDMA and Related Compounds

Chemically, this series of about 150 chemicals stands between mescaline and amphetamine in structure. They exhibit psychotomimetic effects, but are euphoriants at lower dosages. They have been used sequentially since the late 1960s either to avoid legal controls or to achieve "psychedelic drug of the year" status. DOM, also called STP (Serenity, Tranquility, Peace), was superceded by MDA (the Love Drug) which gave way to MDMA (Ecstasy).

This drug series acts over serotonergic neurons like LSD, but MDA produces selective, long-lasting reductions in serotonin brain levels for more than two weeks after the last treatment. In one study, doses of MDA were given every 12 hours for 4 days. The number of serotonin binding sites was reduced, as was the concentration of 5-HIAA, the major metabolite of 5-HT. Degeneration of axons and nerve terminals were found in the hippocampus and striatum, the same areas that sustained a substantial loss of 5-HT activity.

Since MDMA is a closely related analogue of MDA and is experiencing an increase in nonmedical use, it is important to determine whether it also is a neurotoxin. The results of the study show similar serotonin cell degeneration as was noted with MDA.

Opioids

The mechanism of action of the endogenous and exogenous opioids has been reviewed in Chapter 2, pages 36-43.

Cannabis

Despite considerable study, the neurochemical explanation of the mental effects of marijuana remains incomplete. The marked increase in heart rate with lesser elevations of blood pressure associated with orthostatic hypotension could be understood as an adrenergic-mediated effect. This can be prevented by administering the beta adrenergic blocking agent, propranolol. Dopamine release has also been demonstrated.

A decrease in hippocampal cholinergic mechanisms has been observed in some studies, which may explain the defect in immediate recall. Inhibition of prostaglandin synthetase occurs *in vivo* and *in vitro*, but these observations do not clarify the cause of the thought and perceptual alterations associated with THC (the active ingredient in marijuana). A THC receptor has been described, but nonpsychoactive THC analogues also bind to the receptor.

It can be said that the long retention of THC and its active 11-hydroxy-THC metabolite are due to binding in the body's lipid tissues as fatty acid conjugates. The cannabinoids are slowly released back into the bloodstream and are distributed to the brain and other body tissues, eventually being excreted in the urine and feces. Whether the low brain levels of THC that result from the remobilization from body fat in long-term users produce neurobehavioral effects is unknown.

Phencyclidine (PCP)

PCP is a complicated drug. In fact, Osler's dictum about

syphilis can be paraphrased to read: "If you understand PCP, you understand much of neuropsychiatry." It has dopaminergic, adrenergic, serotonergic, cholinergic, GABA-ergic, opioidergic, glutaminergic, and anticholinergic effects. It also has strong membrane effects apart from its neurotransmitter activity.

A basic capability to block the reuptake of the monoamines, and to perhaps increase their synthesis and release into the synapse, accounts for many of phencyclidine's actions. This enhances transmitter effects which sometimes are oppositional. A common property of neuronal action is a selective blockade of K^+ channels, thereby prolonging neuroelectrical transmission and the entry of Ca^{++} into the terminal bouton, which is responsible for increased transmitter release.

The sigma opioid receptor has been identified as one of the two stereospecific binding sites for which PCP has an affinity. This sigma receptor is the recognition site for the psychotomimetic opioids such as cyclazocine, an opioid agonist-antagonist. Naloxone does not block the sigma receptor. An endogenous ligand for the sigma receptor has been identified and called alpha endopyschosin. An antagonist is also known.

Some of the common effects of PCP will be mentioned along with the presumed transmitter responsibility for it, recognizing that very complicated interactions occur.

Dopamine excess may account for the euphoria, stereotyped behavior, and the schizophreniform psychosis. The sigma opioid activity might contribute to the psychosis and the analgesic action. Glutamate could be responsible for the increased strength and the convulsions with adrenergic effects also contributing to the latter symptom. NE activity probably causes the autonomic signs of tachycardia and hypertension and some degree of the hyperactivity. The sedation is either serotonergic, GABA-ergic, or both. The drooling is a cholinergic action.

Sedative-hypnotics

Barbiturates

The barbiturates and related hypnosedatives have a generalized depressant action on the CNS. As with alcohol, an inhibition of neuronal activity from anxiety reduction to coma occurs. The depressant activity is achieved by potentiation of GABA-ergic transmission, a diminished Ca^{++} ion channel activity with a resultant decreased release of neurotransmitters. Glutamate induces depolarizaiton, and its action is reversed by barbiturates, adding to the CNS depression. Since the barbiturates act over GABA transmission, they therefore will add to the effects of benzodiazepines.

It is the increase in Cl^- ion conduction which prevents depolarization, thus preventing neurotransmission, that is crucial in the action of sedative hypnotics. The interaction of Cl^- ion channels, GABA neurons, benzodiazepine receptors, and the barbiturate effect upon this system accounts for what is called tranquilization, or in large doses, sedation or coma.

Benzodiazepines

The benzodiazepines, by virtue of their specific recognition sites, act by potentiating the action of GABA, thus increasing neural inhibition. At present two types of binding sites are known, both adjacent to GABA receptors, and they are found in areas that are consistent with the activity of the benzodiazepine group.

The anxiolytic, the anticonvulsant, and the muscle relaxant capabilities of this group are readily explained by their enhancement of GABA-ergic transmission which dampens monoamine activity.

Anxiety and Panic

Disabling anxiety is a common disorder. Panic attacks or extreme anxiety without an apparent cause occur in two to three percent of the population. Panic episodes can be duplicated in people who experience them by breathing a small amount of carbon dioxide or by receiving a lactic acid solution intravenously. These procedures have in common an increased acidity of the blood. Acidity receptors are present in the brain, and they may be hypersensitive in people susceptible to panic. In anxiety states NE levels may be elevated. Increased NE production may be genetic, environmental, or related to early learning.

The classical anti-anxiety agents, ethanol, bromides, chloral, and paraldehyde, are sedatives with a variety of undesirable effects when used for anxiolytic purposes. Small amounts of the barbiturates were an improvement, but their therapeutic/toxic ratio was low.

The benzodiazepines are the most widely used group of drugs for the treatment of anxiety and insomnia. They have a selective affinity for certain GABA receptors, and many achieve a daytime anxiolytic response without excessive drowsiness. The recognition sites for benzodiazepines are believed to accept an endogenous anxiety-inducing peptide (diazepam binding inhibitor) that induces what is called anxiety. Exogenous site-specific benzodiazepine antagonists are known.

Propranolol (Inderal), a beta-adrenergic antagonist, has been employed to block the peripheral manifestation of anxiety, and therefore to break up the feedback of feelings of tension, tachycardia, etc., from the periphery back into the brain. Busipirone (Buspar) is a new class of anxiolytics that does not act on the GABA receptor. It is said to produce less sedation than the benzodiazepines. Its mechanism of action is unknown.

Alcohol

The acute ingestion of ethanol leads to a fluidization of the neuronal cell membrane. K^+ and Cl^- ion channels are opened, and Na^+ and Ca^- channels close. These changes would lead to CNS depression (hyperpolarization). Catecholamine concentrations are elevated. This can account for the elevation of blood pressure and the increased heart rate often noted. Acute intake produces a coupling of alcohol to adenylate cyclase and stimulates the production of cAMP. During chronic alcohol use, cAMP activity is inhibited. The inhibition is probably due to alcohol's effects on membrane proteins and adenosine. The withdrawal state, which is characterized by excitation of the CNS, is associated with membrane rigidity and a reversal of the ion channel events that occurred during intoxication.

Whether condensation products of acetaldehyde (the first metabolite of alcohol) and one of the biogenic amines are synthesized in the brain into tetrahydroisoquinolines (TIQs) is questionable. Some researchers believe that such events can produce significant amounts of the TIQs and attribute the withdrawal effects to the isoquinolines, which have some structural resemblance to morphine. However, the morphine abstinence syndrome is quite different from the alcohol abstinence syndrome. Barbiturate and alcohol CNS effects are similar, as is their withdrawal symptomatology. This is probably because they both close Cl^- and open Ca^{++} channels during withdrawal.

Volatile Solvents

An array of dozens of volatile solvents are occasionally abused by minors and others who do not have easy access to alcohol. They include industrial fluids that are intentionally inhaled, for example, toluene or gasoline. Butyl and amyl nitrites are sniffed for their euphorogenic and orgasm-enhancing purposes. Anesthetics like ether and nitrous oxide have induced outbreaks of abuse.

The intoxicating action of these volatiles are presumptively due to their cellular membrane effect. They are all lipid soluble and alter the characteristics of the phospholipids embedded within the neuronal membrane. In so doing they interfere with neurotransmission in low doses increasing and in anesthetic doses sharply decreasing it.

Anticholinergic Agents

Many classes of drugs have anticholinergic properties: antipsychotics, antidepressants, antispasmotics, anti-Parkinsonism drugs, antihistamines, and many plants like belladonna. Some of them are abused, for example, scopolamine, amitriptyline (Elavil), trihexyphenidyl (Artane), tripelennamine (Pyribenzamine), and Jimson weed.

Anticholinergic drugs antagonize the action of acetylcholine, particularly at the muscarinic receptors. In the CNS large doses of atropine or other anticholinergic drugs induce a delirium which can be followed by coma and respiratory paralysis. The major effects of the muscarinic cholinergic blocking agents are on the viscera—increasing heart rate, slowing the gastrointestinal tract, reducing gastric secretion, and dilating the pupils.

Nicotine

Nicotine is the addictive agent in tobacco. It is a stimulant to the CNS, producing tremulousness, increased respiration and, in sensitive people, convulsions. Nicotine poisoning causes a depression of the respiratory center. It acts upon the nicotinic receptors of the autonomic nervous system to increase or decrease the release of ACh, depending on the dosage. In addition, it stimulates the release of DA and NE. Animals will self-administer nicotine, but it is much less reinforcing than amphetamine.

Some tolerance develops to nicotine, especially to its gastrointestinal and cardioregulatory effects. Smokers will increase their intake to some specific level and maintain that intake over years. If they substitute a low-nicotine cigarette, they will manipulate their intake to procure their usual dosage of nicotine. Despite being only mildly rewarding, nicotine is a difficult addiction to overcome.

4

The Pharmacotherapy of the Addictions

Treatment of the addictive process requires multiple approaches. In this chapter only the psychochemotherapeutic aspects will be discussed, and only those developed recently will be emphasized.

Opioids

Detoxification

The traditional detoxification medication is methadone administered orally. However, a nonnarcotic has been proposed, in part because it permits immediate patient transfer to opioid antagonist treatment. That drug is clonidine (Catapres), an antihypertensive and alpha$_2$ adrenergic agonist. The principle of clonidine use is that opioids suppress NE locus ceruleus activity. When the narcotic is stopped, a release from inhibitory activity occurs, and an array of symptoms called the withdrawal sickness intervenes. To avoid these uncomfortable symptoms, clonidine is administered, because locus ceruleus adrenergic hyperactivity is counteracted by the inhibitory adrenergic agonist. The actual mechanism consists of an opening of K^+ channels via cAMP and a reduction of locus ceruleus firing.

Theoretically, any opioid could be used to detoxify. Propoxyphene napsylate (Darvon-N) has had a few clinical trials. Nonnarcotics including antispasmotics, analgesics, and sedatives, often in combination, have been utilized for partial relief.

Other drugs and techniques (hypnosis, acupuncture, etc.) have been employed to detoxify heroin-dependent people. Considering the low potency of heroin on the street, it is not surprising that almost everything seems to work. In fact, the therapeutic community Synanon requires "cold turkey" withdrawal utilizing nothing but group support. Alcohol, sleeping pills, and tranquilizers will ameliorate the moderate withdrawal syndromes seen at present.

Maintenance Therapy

The rationale for opioid maintenance is simple. A large number of addicts will not enter or will fail in drug-free programs. Therefore, the addicts and the community benefit from their maintenance on an oral, long-acting, cross tolerance-producing narcotic. The goal is eventual abstinence, but a few methadone-maintained patients have received the drug for 25 years without adverse sequellae.

Methadone is a mu agonist that is given by mouth once daily. A prolonged action form that is effective with three times weekly administration is 1-alpha-acetylmethadol (LAAM). Although not yet available commercially, it has been given to thousands of patients. Some patients prefer methadone, others LAAM.

Other opioids have, to a lesser extent, been employed as maintenance agents. Opium is used in a few countries. Codeine could theoretically be used. Buprenorphine (Buprenex) is a partial mu agonist with some antagonistic features. It is about 30 times more potent than morphine and can suppress signs of morphine withdrawal in abstinent patients. However, buprenorphine precipitates withdrawal in actively using opioid-dependent individuals. Withdrawal from buprenorphine is moderate to absent, and physical dependence may not occur. It has been suggested as a maintenance or detoxification agent, especially when detoxification from methadone maintenance is required.

It would be incorrect to assume that heroin maintenance is practiced in Great Britain, as some people believe. According to the most recent Home Office report (December 31, 1986) only two percent of heroin addicts at the governmental treatment centers are being given heroin. The rest receive methadone, and a few are given dipipanone. The disadvantage of heroin as a maintenance agent is that 4 to 6 injections a day must be administered, with all the related dangers of the diseases of unsterility. An ideal maintenance drug should be long-acting, effective orally, inexpensive, and not be capable of being injected. Heroin does not fulfill any of these requirements.

Narcotic Antagonists

Naltrexone (Trexan), a long-acting, pure opioid antagonist, has been available for those who require a chemical deterrent to remain abstinent. Naltrexone binds competitively to mu and kappa receptors, preventing detoxified opioid addicts from experiencing the reinforcing euphoric effects of exogenous narcotics. The possibility also exists that when a number of injections of heroin go unreinforced, heroin-seeking behavior will eventually stop.

The antagonist, naloxone (Narcan), can be used as a test to ascertain whether opioids have recently been used. The rapid, but short-acting, naloxone will produce either evidence of withdrawal or, at least, pupillary dilation if opioids are displaced from their receptors. If they are, naltrexone treatment should be withheld until opioids have been eliminated from their brain binding sites.

Naltrexone stimulates the secretion of LH, FSH and ACTH, and it inhibits the release of prolactin and growth hormones. Although naltrexone is a long-acting drug, a still greater prolongation of activity would be advantageous. A sustained release form of naltrexone has been prepared consisting of biodegradable naltrexone beads implanted subcutaneously. Plasma naltrexone levels were maintained for one month in amounts sufficient to block a morphine challenge. Such a polymer plastic preparation may have value in the treatment of selected patients who may "forget" to take their oral medication.

Sedative-hypnotics, Tranquilizers and Alcohol

These drugs manifest cross tolerance and cross dependence to each other. Therefore they can be considered together insofar as treatment is concerned, with the exception that alcohol dependence requires additional measures. They are all CNS depressants, and most of them open Cl^- ion channels, increasing intracellular negativity (hyperpolarization) and preventing depolarization.

Detoxification

With a dependent person it is usually necessary to reduce the daily dosage gradually, sometimes in a hospital setting. Decremental detoxification is required to avoid convulsions or a toxic psychosis because abrupt discontinuance of CNS depressants lowers the convulsive threshold and releases hallucinatory-confusional states. Any CNS depressant can be employed in the gradual reduction of dosage, but it is conventional to use a benzodiazepine, such as chlordiazepoxide (Librium), for alcohol detoxification and phenobarbital for sedative-hypnotic detoxification. These are long-acting drugs and require fewer doses per day to maintain blood levels.

Deterrent Agents

During the sober interval, some alcoholics have been given disulfiram (Antabuse) or other drugs that interfere with the oxidation of acetaldehyde. The rationale for such medication is that acetaldehyde, the first metabolite of alcohol, is a toxic substance that produces flushing, respiratory difficulties, nausea, and hypotension. When the enzyme aldehyde dehydrogenase is blocked by disulfiram, the breakdown of acetaldehyde to acetate is reduced to the point that blood acetaldehyde levels increase and noxious effects are produced. The alcohol-Antabuse reaction may be mild, but it can be life-endangering if large amounts of both drugs are ingested.

Aversion Techniques

Pairing the drinking of alcoholic beverages with an emetic like apomorphine or emetine can evoke a conditioned avoidance response to ethanol. The use of aversive stimuli to make the act of drinking sickening has waned, but is still widely used in the Soviet Union and other Eastern European countries. Apomorphine is a dopamine agonist and has been tried as an anticraving medication in less than emetic doses. Pairing alcohol intake with a moderately painful electric shock does not seem to work well.

Amethystic Agents

The acceleration of the sobering-up process has been sought after for a long time. Many folk remedies have been proposed, including cups made of amethyst which were supposed to prevent drunkenness. Oxygen inhalations and nutritional supplements have been used. Increasing the metabolism of alcohol is difficult, and it has not been established that the currently available intoxication preventers or reducers are effective.

A different approach to amethystics has been tried in rodents. It is known that alcohol acts on the GABA receptor. It diminishes firing by allowing Cl^- influx and hyperpolarization of the neuronal membrane. A benzodiazepine antagonist is known that selectively diminishes or abolishes drunken behavior by reducing the GABA-ergic Cl^- influx. Taken before alcohol, it is supposed to prevent intoxication. Taken after alcohol it has revived stuporous rats within minutes. The benzodiazepine in question, R015-4513, is being tried in humans. Although blood alcohol levels do not fall, intoxicated behavior improves. Effects last for 20 to 30 minutes and a longer-acting analogue is being sought.

Other Pharmacotherapies

Lithium carbonate has been tried in an attempt to reduce alcohol consumption. The tricyclic antidepressants have been tested during the abstinent phase in nondepressed patients. Neither treatment seems particularly effective except in patients with manic-depressive disorders.

The benzodiazepines have an established value in dealing with severe anxiety during the postintoxication state. Beta adrenergic blockers also ameliorate the tension and occasional panic of the alcohol withdrawal syndrome.

Cocaine and Amphetamines

The pharmacotherapy of cocaine dependence is of lesser importance than personal, interpersonal, and environmental readjustment manipulations.

Detoxification

These drugs require no gradual reduction, since potentially serious withdrawal effects, except depression, will not occur with abrupt discontinuance. In fact, a program of slow removal of a central stimulant is contraindicated because time, and perhaps the patient, may be lost to treatment. Analgesics and sedatives are sometimes needed for the first few days.

What is called the detoxification period for stimulants consists of physical and psychological repair, motivational enhancement, relapse prevention, and planning for further management.

Maintenance

Although no strong support for a stimulant maintenance therapy exists, a few clinical trials have been considered or performed. Methylphenidate was tried for cocaine dependence without success, because the development of tolerance was so rapid that large doses had to be administered without affecting relapse back to cocaine. Pemoline (Cylert) is a less stimulating stimulant and has hardly been tried in the cocaine-dependent person. Some evidence exists that synthetic local anesthetics like procaine and lidocaine are reinforcing and might be able to replace cocaine use. From what is known of stimulant pharmacology, maintenance therapy would be a dubious addition to our therapeutic options.

The use of cocaine itself as a maintenance agent is irrational, even if given orally. Dosage control would be a major problem, and tolerance to the euphoria will defeat attempts at stabilization. Quite properly, no one has yet proposed cocaine maintenance as a treatment.

Agonists

If the cocaine hunger is due to a dopamine deficiency during the early abstinent state, then it would be reasonable to try noneuphoriant dopamine agonists. This has been done in some preliminary studies.

Bromocriptine (Parlodel) is a dopamine agonist that has been found to reduce symptoms associated with the cocaine "crash," and when given for a few weeks after drug use is stopped, it seems to diminish craving. These have been open studies with the blind investigations not yet published. Such a therapeutic agent might also be expected to ameliorate the anhedonia that can last for weeks after cocaine has been discontinued.

Amantadine (Symmetrel) is another dopamine agonist that is being studied in clinical trials. Claims of reduction of episodes of craving have been put forward. Controlled studies will be needed to confirm the initial impressions.

Precursors

Tryptophan

Since 5-HT does not pass the blood-brain barrier, its precursor, tryptophan, has been given during the postcocaine state to increase 5-HT stores and to obtain sleep. Most of the ingested tryptophan is used to build proteins and for other purposes, but some does reach the brain. It may have an effect on 5-HT depletion, but controlled studies have not been done.

Tyrosine

As a precursor of dopamine and norepinephrine, the amino acid tyrosine may be a rational approach. Both positive and negative clinical reports can be found in the literature. One thing is certain: in order to produce an effect, doses of up to 10 grams a day will be needed. Like tryptophan, only a small amount of the tyrosine consumed reaches the brain.

L-dopa (Levodopa)

Since L-dopa is the immediate precursor of DA and NE, it would be expected that L-dopa or carbidopa (Sinemet) would be used to correct any DA depletion. However, L-dopa is not mentioned as a precursor replenishment agent in articles on cocaine.

The notion that DA and NE availability are diminished as a result of excessive cocaine use is reasonable but incompletely proved. Changes in receptor function are just as likely.

Euphoria Blockers

Lithium

Lithium has been tried as a blocking agent to prevent cocaine euphoria. Anti-euphoriant effects have not been found with any consistency. The drug must be monitored for blood levels; otherwise toxicity may occur. The difficulties in administering lithium carbonate and the mixed results do not recommend it as a euphoria blocker, but it has a definite value in the treatment of a cocaine abuser who also is manic. If lithium worked, it would be by inhibiting depolarization and the Ca^{++} dependent release of DA and NE. While such events might be desirable during the intoxicated period, it would not be advantageous during the withdrawal phase.

Dopamine Antagonists

A straightforward way to deal with cocaine dependence would appear to be the use of dopamine antagonists. They should block euphoria and break the cycle of positive reinforcement that demands further cocaine acquisition and usage. More than a dozen DA receptor antagonists are marketed. The high potency neuroleptics might be preferred, probably in small doses. No major research effort has been launched to test the hypotheses that neuroleptics like haloperidol (Haldol) protect against further cocaine intake. It may be that since these agents have unpleasant side effects and are not harmless, this line of investigation has not been pursued. Still, for patients who strongly want to get off cocaine or amphetamines, but who are not sure that the urge to use the stimulants could be resisted, a trial using modest doses might be indicated.

Antidepressants

The tricyclic antidepressants (TCAs) are used for two reasons following cocaine discontinuance: for depression and to reduce the drive to use the drug. The TCAs are effective, but it is common for the postcocaine depression to last no more than three weeks even without treatment. In some cases the credit given to the TCAs may not be deserved. TCAs that are secondary amines like desipramine (Norpramine) and block NE reuptake, as well as tertiary amines like imipramine (Tofranil) that block 5-HT reuptake, are effective in dealing with postcocaine depressions.

A number of claims have been made that craving is reduced by TCAs. The rationale seems to be that TCAs produce effects opposite to that existing in the postcocaine CNS circuitry. Normalization of the catecholaminergic circuitry may occur, decreasing anhedonia and dysphoria, and therefore reducing drug hunger. The hypothesis has not yet been stringently tested.

Phencyclidine (PCP)

Detoxification is unnecessary for PCP intoxication. In fact, procedures have been used to encourage the excretion of the drug. Since it is attracted to acid ions, infusions of dilute hydrochloric acid and ammonium chloride have been used till the acidity of the urine is down to a pH of 5.0. In milder cases oral ascorbic acid or cranberry juice have been given. Continuous gastric suction will remove large amounts of phencyclidine because it is attracted to the hydrochloric acid in the stomach. These ion-trapping techniques have dangers and must be carefully monitored because a respiratory and metabolic acidosis may also exist.

5

The Genetics of Substance Abuse

In considering the complexities of the process of becoming drug dependent, the social, psychological, and cultural factors must be acknowledged. However, there is mounting evidence of a genetic component to the compulsive use of mind-altering substances. Alcoholism will be emphasized because it is the drug that has received the most research attention. Brief mention of what is known about the genetic loading for other drugs will be included.

Alcohol

A perennial question that has concerned scholars of the human-alcohol interaction has been: "Why is it that two people with approximately similar personalities, with similar sociocultural backgrounds, levels of stress, etc., will have entirely divergent drinking patterns? One will drink moderately for a lifetime and the other will become an alcoholic." In many instances it might be found that the alcoholic had first-degree relatives who also had destructive drinking patterns. In itself, a history of familial alcoholism is no proof that it is an inherited disease. Early rearing practices may have shaped the drinking behavior of the child in the direction of heavy drinking and subsequent addiction to alcohol.

So the ancient observation that drunkenness runs in families is insufficient evidence to say that it is inherited.

Animal Studies

A normal distribution curve exists for ethanol drinking behavior within any species. By mating the animals with a predeliction to drink, and by also breeding animals who refuse to consume alcohol, after a few generations two strains will emerge. One strain will drink willingly, preferring alcohol solutions to water; the other will not drink at all, and in fact, will avoid alcohol. Such rat lineages have been developed and are used in the research on alcohol-seeking behavior. The rats in the drinking group work to secure an alcohol solution in preference to water and will become physically addicted to ethanol. They will go into the DTs if they are abruptly withdrawn from their preferred potion. Lower brain levels of 5-HT and 5-HIAA are found in various areas like the hippocampus and cortex in those rats who preferred alcohol to water even before exposure to alcohol. The nondrinking line will abstain if offered alcohol or will taste it on rare occasions.

The alcoholic rats were drinking for the purpose of becoming intoxicated, not because they liked the taste or smell of the alcohol. This was proved in experiments in which two flavored solutions were proffered. If rats drank solution "A," they would get a dose of alcohol instilled into their stomachs. If they chose flavor "B," the stomach tube would contain water. Alcoholic rats quickly learned that "A" was their choice. After a while, the flavors were switched so that "B" would lead to intragastric alcohol and "A" to water. The inebriate rats switched to solution "B".

In another study, when water was substituted for alcohol solution, the rats decreased their consumption markedly, but when alcohol was restored, the alcohol-preferring rats started their heavy drinking again. It should be noted that water was available in their cages at all times. The nonalcoholic rats took very little of the solution that contained alcohol.

It seems evident from these studies and others that a strain of alcohol-seeking rats can be bred who selectively prefer large amounts of alcohol for the effect it has on their brains—namely intoxication, sedation, and sleep. The low intake group of rats exposed to identical conditions imbibed no more than the equivalent of one drink. This series of investigations provide strong support for the role of genetic factors in the development of alcoholism. Its application to the human species is direct, except for the fact that humans are not bred to be alcoholics or nonalcoholics, but have a variable genetic potential to become alcoholics. If abstinent and dipsomaniacal rats can be bred, this must mean that differences in the genetic structure of the two groups exist. We are not yet aware of the biochemical substrate of the genetic disturbance that produces inherited approach behavior to alcohol.

Human Studies

Adoption Studies

A number of strategies have been tried in an effort to demonstrate that humans also show evidence for a genetic predisposition to become alcoholics. When a large number of adopted male children of alcoholics were compared to the adopted male children of nonalcoholics, it was found that children of alcoholics were three times as likely to develop alcoholism. The drinking practices of the foster parents were not a significant variable. Dependence on alcohol was also more severe and began at an earlier age. Alcohol abuse in the biological mothers and fathers produced children who were significantly more likely to become alcoholics than in the nonalcoholic parental group.

When hospitalized alcoholics were surveyed, more than three times as many had an alcoholic biological parent as those in a control group consisting of their nonalcoholic half siblings. This indicated that the parent not related to either sibling was contributing a genetic predisposition to either become or not to become an alcoholic.

The Scandinavian adoption studies have been convincing in furthering the idea of a genetic factor in alcoholism. In one such study children were adopted before the age of three. Both their biological and their adoptive parents were meticulously studied. Some of the conclusions derived included the following:

1. In some alcoholic families only the male children tend to develop alcoholism; in others both sexes are vulnerable.

2. Father-son or mother-daughter inheritance poses a greater risk than father-daughter transmission. Mother-son inheritance produces significantly more alcoholism compared to nonalcoholic biological parents.

3. The degree of alcoholism in parents was a significant factor in the degree of children's inherited severity of alcoholism.

4. Alcohol abuse (problem drinking) in the adoptive parents was not related to alcohol abuse in the adopted children.

5. Two types of genetic predispositions could be discerned. More frequently, the gene or genes for alcoholism are present, but do not become manifest unless an environmental loading is also present (such as low income or if the adoptive father had an unskilled-type job). Another less frequent type of inherited susceptibility occurs in father-son dyads and is ordinarily more malignant in nature. The father-son inheritance is apparently not dependent on environmental stressors.

In a study of combat and noncombat veterans it was found

that two-thirds of the veterans who had not experienced combat had no alcohol problems, while two-thirds of the combat veterans did have problems with alcohol. The severity of the alcoholism in the latter group correlated directly with the amount of combat exposure. This study seems to emphasize again the influence of environmental factors, or at least the importance of environment in making alcoholism manifest in those with an inborn vulnerability.

Twin Studies

A number of investigations into twins have generally supported the idea of the genetic contribution to alcoholism. Identical twins share 100% of their genes; fraternal twins share 50% of their genetic makeup. If alcoholism is a genetically influenced disorder, the rate of concordance in alcoholism should be higher in the identical (one egg) than in same-sex fraternal (two egg) twins. This has been demonstrated. When one identical twin is alcoholic, the other has a 55% chance of being alcoholic. When one fraternal twin is alcoholic, the concordance rate is 28%. The fact that twins with identical genetic composition have a 55% concordance rate and not 100% illustrates that other factors, such as the personal environment, are involved in about half of those who carry the gene for alcohol addiction.

Therefore, inevitable alcoholism is not a viable concept, even for those whose families are replete with alcoholics. But such studies help in the identification of high-risk groups and have a value in prevention.

The fact that a number of close relatives in a family were alcoholic does not mean that the daughters and sons will inevitably succumb to the same disorder. It does mean that the probability is greater—that what is inherited is an increased vulnerability. Knowing this, the vulnerable person must make a decision about drinking alcoholic beverages. The best decision would be to abstain.

It is interesting that the risk of alcoholism in the relatives of alcoholics changes between generations, dependent upon changes in social usage. As alcohol becomes more available and acceptable, the expression of the genetic risk factors increases. This finding again provides evidence that both genetic and environmental factors are necessary for the development of alcoholism.

An enormous variability in sensitivity to alcohol exists. People are known who can drink consistently for long periods and remain quite alert or, at least, not grossly intoxicated. In body sway tests following exposure to alcohol, those with a positive family history of alcoholism are less affected than those with a negative family history. Persons from alcoholic families also feel the effects of alcohol less. It may be that the relative resistance to alcohol makes those with an inherited vulnerability less able to know when to stop drinking.

Certain individuals have an adverse reaction to a single drink. These individuals have what can be called "the Oriental flush syndrome," which is noted in more than half of those of Mongolian ancestry. A flush over the chest and face, tachycardia, and a lowered blood pressure constitute the major features of the syndrome, although rarely a shock-like condition can develop. It is an unpleasant condition and may deter heavy drinking. Some observers believe that the syndrome accounts for the lower prevalence of alcoholism among Japanese, Korean, and Chinese people. However, American Indians also flush as much as the Mongolian populations they left in Asia, and they have a very serious problem with alcoholism. This indicates that an unpleasant reaction to alcohol is no absolute protection from drinking problems.

Hypersensitive responses to alcohol are due to an accumulation of acetaldehyde. This can be caused by a too-rapid transformation of alcohol to acetaldehyde by alcohol dehydrogenase. It is more likely the result of an accumulation of acetaldehyde caused by an inefficient variant of the enzyme aldehyde dehydrogenase, which causes buildup of the quite toxic acetaldehyde. The same phenomenon is witnessed when alcohol and disulfiram (Antabuse) are taken together. The drug prevents aldehyde dehydrogenase from degrading acetaldehyde to acetate. So the alcohol-Antabuse reaction is essentially an acetaldehyde intoxication, and it resembles the inherited Oriental flush syndrome. Other enzymes also are involved in the catabolism of alcohol. In addition to the variants of alcohol and acetaldehyde dehydrogenase, catalase and the microsomal ethanol oxidizing system become active when large amounts of alcohol are consumed. All of these enzymes evolved for the purpose of detoxifying the ounce or so of ethanol generated daily by intestinal fermentation and absorbed via the intestine.

Although variant types of alcohol-metabolizing systems are inherited and may deter certain populations from overimbibing, these differences may not be as important as other factors in explaining what is genetically transmitted in a family's vulnerability to alcohol.

It is evident that genetics is not destiny. Environmental, personal, and cultural factors exert an important influence on whether the genetically loaded person becomes an alcoholic. These factors also determine whether individuals with a built-in aversive response to alcohol, including many Asian people, will be protected from becoming alcoholic. Those who have no genetic loading whatsoever to alcohol cannot be assured that they are immune to becoming alcoholic. It may be that a majority of alcoholics have no inherited vulnerability. Their condition may be caused by a vain effort to treat their depression, anxiety, inability to cope, or other problems with beverage alcohol. Or they may have been trained by their culture, family, or friends to drink dysfunctionally.

Theories

If gene changes are involved in alcohol dependence, then the changes must be expressed in some neurochemical alteration. Various possibilities exist, and some research support for each theory is available. These hypotheses will be noted, recognizing that none is conclusive.

The Membrane Theory

It has been noted that alcohol makes the neuronal membrane less viscous, therefore more fluid. The altered viscosity of the membranes interferes with the action of neurotransmitters, the membrane proteins and their enzymes. Adenosine triphosphate (ATP) and its enzyme adenylate cyclase activate the ion pump that regulates the inflow and outflow of Na^+ and K^+ through the membrane pores. It is speculated that a genetic predisposition would occur if the form of adenylate cyclase which is inherited could alter the reactivity of the ion pumps.

The Neurotransmitter Hypothesis

Research has shown that alcohol inhibits Ca^{++} uptake into the presynaptic neuron, thereby interfering with the release of NE, DA, 5-HT and GABA. Chronic use encourages NE and DA release. Mice that were bred to be resistant to the behavioral effects of alcohol had little change in dopamine release. GABA receptor sites are increased during alcohol intake and decreased during withdrawal. Since GABA is an inhibitory transmitter, these effects are consistent with sedation during active use and seizure activity during withdrawal. A predisposition to alcoholism might be due to genetic variations in neurotransmitter release and receptivity.

The Tetrahydroisoquinoline (TIQ) Model

When acetaldehyde and a catecholamine condense, the resulting structure resembles morphine and has a morphine-like action. These are TIQs. This finding led to the assumption that alcohol and the opioids may share a common addictive mechanism. There is some evidence that TIQs in minute amounts are formed in the brain without alcohol, but they are present in greater quantities in alcoholics than nonalcoholics. Could a genetic defect in alcoholics reduce their capacity to metabolize acetaldehyde, resulting in the overproduction of TIQs?

It is unlikely that alcohol and opioids share a common addiction mechanism. The withdrawal syndromes of alcohol and opioids are very different. The levels of TIQs achieved during the acute alcoholic state are not impressive. Nevertheless, it is an interesting speculation.

The Reinforcement Hypothesis

The possible inheritance of mechanisms in the brain that are unusually responsive to the reinforcing effects of alcohol has been suggested. In other words, the intoxicated state is more rewarding to potential alcoholics than to others. The initial phase of drinking is stimulating and may be more pleasurable to some drinkers. The subsequent punishing, dysphoric phase of intoxication may not be too well remembered by heavy drinkers because they have blackouts or have other memory defects. Alcohol may be used by predisposed alcoholics for reasons similar to those who use cocaine, amphetamine, or heroin compulsively. Alcohol provides more euphoria for them than other people obtain from alcohol. If this is so, then dopaminergic and adrenergic mechanisms are involved, perhaps also the opioid peptides.

A variant of this theory is that alcoholics have a congenital inability to enjoy ordinary life pleasures. Perhaps they have an inborn deficiency of receptors at the reward centers or a deficiency in dopaminergic neurons to those reward centers. Alcohol provides them with a way to make up for their reward system malfunction. They obtain so much more gratification from ethanol than nonalcoholics that they become locked into its use.

Still another possibility is that the alcoholic has inherited a CNS with a low tolerance for frustration, stress, or anxiety. Therefore their suffering is greater even though their existence is not necessarily more stressful. Alcohol serves as an antianxiety agent, relieving the unpleasurable moods and the suffering.

Markers of Alcoholism

If alcoholism is a genetic disease, then some evidence of it must exist even before the first drink is taken. The search for physiological or biochemical characteristics that would be associated with alcoholism is ongoing in a variety of laboratories.

Physiological Markers

In some studies, event-related potentials (ERPs) are derived from the brain in an effort to find unique electrical events following auditory or visual stimulation. In one study the sons of fathers who were diagnosed alcoholics were compared to the sons of nonalcoholic fathers. Significant differences in the P3 waves of the ERP were found in the sons of the alcoholic fathers, whether or not alcohol was administered during the experiment. This finding has been confirmed by others. The P3 wave showed lower amplitudes in the sons of alcoholic fathers even though the sons had never used alcohol previously. In addition, they had longer reaction times and had fewer correct responses on psychological testing.

A number of neuromuscular coordination disorders were found to be associated with an increased risk for becoming alcoholic. For example, essential (familial) tremor is likely to be associated with alcoholism, and the relatives of alcoholics are more likely to have essential tremor than relatives of nonalcoholics. Static ataxia (difficulty in the ability to maintain equilibrium while standing with feet together) is also more likely to be associated with paternal alcoholism than in a matched control group.

Enzyme Markers

The processing of alcohol through acetaldehyde to acetate is performed by hepatic alcohol- and aldehyde-dehydrogenases. Some 20 varieties of alcohol dehydrogenases are known, some of them inactive. Whether the gene for alcoholism is expressed in some variant of the dehydrogenases remains obscure.

Biologic markers for alcoholism are described, but these result from the effects of the drug rather than from its causes. A representative sample of alcohol-caused markers would include the red blood cell mean corpuscular volume, serum uric acid, specific liver function tests, and increased erythrocyte fragility.

Drugs Other Than Alcohol

The search for evidence of genetic relationships for drugs other than alcohol is much sparser than for alcohol. Although correlations between drug-using youths and their parents exist, this could be as readily explainable on the basis of social elements as on genetic ones.

The opioids constitute the best of the poor evidence that

any one drug class may have an inherited contribution to its addiction potential. Rats and mice with high or with low morphine solution drinking propensities have been bred.

The most interesting possibility, but theoretical rather than proven, is that inherited differences in the neuropeptides and their receptors may account for some of the variance in opioid dependence. Data to support such a hypothesis do not exist, but it will be a logical area to research. People have a wide variety of pain thresholds. It is possible that the variation is caused by differences in endorphin levels or in the number or sensitivity of their receptors. Rare cases of an inborn insensitivity to pain are recorded in the scientific literature. Do such people have congenital hyperendorphinosis?

Other concepts include the possibility that no drug-specific genetic vulnerability exists, but that addiction proneness is what can be inherited. Addiction proneness would be manifested by a lowered ability to endure stress or affective disorders, a sociopathic mode of interacting with life or a lack of future orientation. Personality disturbances of this sort make people more likely to become overinvolved in drugs as an attempt at self-treatment, or they may lack the ability to perceive the long-term consequences of their drug usage.

6

Imaging the Brain

Attempts to understand the structure and function of the living brain are ancient, antedating by centuries the first organized efforts of the 19th century phrenologists. It was their hypothesis that the conformation of the skull was indicative of mental faculties and traits of character. Until recently, efforts to gain access to the brain were either indirect or intrusive. Spinal fluid, blood, and urine were analyzed in an effort to ascertain cerebral metabolism. Electroencephalograms could measure summated brain wave patterns from circumscribed areas, but "eyeballing" the tracing lost much of the information that computers now provide. Pneumoencephalograms required the injection of air into the spinal fluid after some fluid had been removed. Cerebral angiography consisted of the injection of a contrast dye to visualize the cerebrovascular system. Some of these procedures were not innocuous. Brain biopsies can be injurious. They can also misinform, because the brain, unlike the liver and kidney, has a regional variability in its chemistry. Skull films retain some diagnostic value but do not compare in clarity with the new imaging procedures.

Recent technological advances have provided an array of instrumentation that gives access to details of structural, electrical, and biochemical information that was impossible to obtain only a decade ago.

The following procedures will be discussed: computed tomography (CT), also called computerized axial tomography (CAT); spectral EEG imaging; positron emission tomography (PET) and single photon tomography; regional cerebral blood flow (rCBF); nuclear magnetic resonance (NMR), also magnetic resonance imaging (MRI); brain electrical activity mapping (BEAM); and magnetoencephalography (MEG).

Computed Tomography (CT)

Utilizing x-ray techniques, CT is able to take pictures of various slices of the head. The brain tissue is visualized almost as clearly as seen in a postmortem section. X-rays penetrate the slice, and contrast depends on the specific gravity of the tissue. Occasionally, a scan utilizing radioactive iodine is used to provide additional contrast. Since their introduction in 1973, CT scans have had a marked impact on neuropsychiatry. Although widely used in the diagnosis of structural defects, it has also been employed for diseases like schizophrenia and the dementias.

Some examples of neuropsychiatric conditions that have been identified by CT include:

Atrophy of diffuse or specific brain structures

Hematomas, hygromas and abscesses

Infarctions, thromboses and hemorrhages

Calcifications and foreign bodies

Normal pressure hydrocephalus

Tumors and cysts

In schizophrenic states, CT has the potential to assist in the diagnosis of Type II, or negative, schizophrenic conditions (those with evidence of regression, withdrawal and hypoactivity). Many such patients carry a clinical diagnosis of undifferentiated or simple schizophrenia. On CT, lateral and third ventricular enlargement with cortical and cerebellar atrophy correlates with the negative symptoms. Acute or paranoid schizophrenics do not show atrophy. Neuropsychological impairment, poor premorbid adjustment, and poor response to treatment are associated with enlarged ventricles.

In another study the lateral ventricular enlargement was significantly greater in schizophrenics than in their well siblings and in a control group. Ventricular size did not differentiate schizophrenics with negative versus positive symptoms, however. It may be that chronicity is an important variable in ventricular enlargement and cerebral atrophy.

When sequential CT scans are taken shortly after abstinence in chronic alcoholics and are repeated at monthly intervals, reversibility of ventricular enlargement (atrophy) can be measured over time. This does not occur in those who relapse. The reversibility can be correlated with neuropsychological testing. Alcoholics show a greater degree of cerebral atrophy than age-matched controls with a variety of neurological diseases.

Spectral EEG Imaging

Arrays of 64 to 128 electrodes can sample the entire cranium and its contents by utilizing a flexible helmet attached to a computer. Space-occupying lesions, the epilepsies, scars, and the effects of certain drugs upon the brain are identifiable. Spectral analysis provides averaged amplitudes for each of the major brain wave frequencies: alpha, beta, delta, and theta for each area subtended. Increases in slow wave (delta) activity have been identified in some untreated schizophrenics.

When a brief visual or auditory signal is provided, the specific response to that stimulus can be recorded from the appropriate brain area. This evoked potential response has been fairly well studied. It has been found that the children of alcoholics have a diminished C_3 wave on the evoked potential even when they have not yet become involved in alcohol. Matched controls from nonalcoholic families do not show this abnormality. If confirmed, this could represent a marker for the genetic vulnerability to become an alcoholic.

In the dementias, a marked slowing of the EEG frequencies are found. Spectral analysis is capable of mapping the brain topographically and providing ratios of the various waves. In dementia of the Alzheimer type, a low delta/theta wave ratio can be identified in the left temporal area. In multi-infarct dementia, theta activity is excessive. Dementia of the Alzheimer type affects cortical areas while multi-infarct dementia can involve both cortex and subcortex.

Positron Emission Tomography (PET)

The PET instrumentation captures and records gamma rays emitted from the slice of tissue that is targeted. The amount of radiation is quantitated and displayed in coded color.

The tracing and quantification of blood movements, diffusion of oxygen and carbon dioxide, and the metabolism of endogenous products from precursor to metabolite can be accomplished by measuring the movement and the reaction rate of the labeled substrate. The tracer is present in such small amounts that it does not interfere with the chemical or physiological processes involved.

Since labeled glucose is rapidly metabolized in the brain, it is customary to use an analogue, 2-deoxy-glucose radio-labeled with ^{18}C or ^{14}C. It does not undergo glucolysis during the time required for PET measurements. The positron emitting isotopes have short half-lives. Therefore, it is possible to perform a series of studies during one session to follow the changes in drug concentration or induced alterations of biochemical or behavioral processes. When the pathways of glucose metabolism are being studied, it is customary to selectively label the carbon atoms in a number of positions.

With PET, measurement of normal and abnormal cerebral

physiology has become possible. Since altered neurochemistry precedes alterations of neuroanatomy, earlier diagnosis becomes possible. A more rational psychochemotherapy becomes feasible when information about the location and duration of drugs is known.

The PET technique includes the use of other labeled compounds. These may be ^{11}C, ^{13}N, ^{15}O or ^{18}F (as a hydrogen substitute). These compounds all have a short half-life and decay by emitting positrons that then combine with electrons to produce gamma rays. These rays penetrate the skull and brain and can be readily detected outside the head. Essentially, every naturally occurring brain chemical can be identified through use of the radioisotopes mentioned. Hundreds of biochemicals have already been labeled, including some by isotopes of Fe, Na, K, P and I.

The accomplishments of PET during the few years of its existence are truly remarkable. Cerebral blood volume, blood flow, and pH are routine procedures. The transport and metabolism of oxygen, glucose, amino acids, fatty acids, and proteins have been measured. The precursors, the neurotransmitters and their metabolites, including dopamine, acetylcholine, epinephrine, norepinephrine, opioids and serotonin, can be scanned. Drugs like the stimulants, anticonvulsants, antidepressants and antipsychotics have been traced. Emotionally loaded interviews, the various stages of sleep, and creative thinking all have fairly characteristic PET maps.

In addition to the extensive use of PET for measuring oxygen and glucose transport and metabolism and blood flow and volume, it is becoming possible to learn the kinetics of protein and amino acid synthesis and breakdown and neurotransmitter-receptor relationships.

While CT and NMR can provide information about the structure of the brain, PET is capable of assessing the functional organization of the brain in a dynamic fashion. Functional imaging ordinarily provides early, larger, and more diversified alterations than the anatomic techniques. This is so because of the enormous interconnections that exist within the brain. What may be seen as a focal lesion on CT may involve assemblies of distant neuronal bundles on PET.

Both nondisease and disease states are amenable to study by PET. Normal human functioning and the mental correlations of thought, emotion, sensation, and the resulting behavior can be analyzed by nonintrusive methods as never before. Some examples can be cited. When a visual stimulus was presented, an average of a 28% increase in glucose utilization in the visual cortex occurred. Auditory stimulation evoked a 17 to 25% increase in the auditory cortex in the temporal lobe. When cognitive tasks were performed, glucose utilization increases varied from 11 to 37% in the frontal cortex. Activation of the hippocampi occurred when memory retrieval was required. Motor tasks produced an 18% increase in glucose utilization in the motor cortex. Hearing speech primarily activated the left auditory cortex, while hearing music predominantly activated the right auditory cortex in right-handed people. Simultaneous language and music activated both hemispheres. Tones, as expected, activated the right hemisphere. When the task was to compare two sounds for similarities or differences, the right side was used. However, if visual imagery was used to solve the task, the left hemisphere was employed.

It is now possible to visualize the neurotransmitter receptor system at work. When ^{11}C methylspiperone, a neuroleptic, is injected, it will bind to D_2 and $5\text{-}HT_2$ receptors. The labeled ligand will bind strongly in the caudate and putamen of the basal ganglia known to contain large numbers of D_2 receptors. In another instance, ^{14}C carfentanyl, a mu opioid agonist, bound to mu receptors in the thalamus, basal ganglia, frontal cortex, and pituitary gland. The density of mu receptors can be estimated in this manner. When naloxone, a mu antagonist, is administered, it blocks the labeled carfentanyl's access to the receptor. The PET scan shows no binding whatsoever when the antagonist is present.

Alcohol affects neuronal function by altering the mechanisms by which information is transmitted. The energy source for neuronal transmission is glucose. The utilization of glucose or its analogue, 2-deoxy-glucose, has been studied in various parts of the brain in order to try to understand where alcohol may exert its activity. Ethanol withdrawal (the DTs) is accompanied by a 25% increase in cerebral oxygen and glucose consumption. Glucose uptake in the frontal-sensory-motor cortex is 150% above the level in controls. In the cerebellar vermis it is 130% higher than controls. Glucose is utilized in twice the amount ordinarily used in the mamillary body, an area of the brain involved in Korsakoff's (alcoholic) psychosis. Korsakoff's psychosis is due to thiamine deficiency, with alcohol a frequent cause, because of the malnutrition and the increased thiamine requirements in the metabolism of alcohol.

PET imaging reveals symmetrical midline alterations in the alcoholic brain along the floor of the ventricles and in the cortex. An abnormal glucose uptake, especially in the frontal cortex, has been found on PET. The finding can lead to earlier identification of the cerebral disorder and to an enhanced ability to evaluate therapeutic efforts when serial studies are used.

Some examples of how PET has been applied clinically include the following:

1. Depression is manifested by decreased glucose utilization in the frontal cortex, more in the left hemisphere.

2. Multiple infarct dementia is associated with multiple areas of cortical and subcortical structures with decreased glucose utilization.

3. Alzheimer's disease is characterized by di-

minished glucose utilization in frontal, temporal and parietal lobes.

4. Huntington's disease. Not only do clinically positive patients have decreased glucose utilization of the caudate and putamen (extrapyramidal areas controlling fine movement), but asymptomatic relatives at risk may be recognized by the presence of a depressed glucose utilization in these structures.

5. Complex partial epilepsy. Glucose utilization is enormously increased in the area during the seizure and decreased elsewhere in the brain. Between seizures glucose utilization is markedly diminished in the ictal area. After successful treatment, the lowered glucose utilization may return to normal.

6. In bipolar affective disorder, glucose utilization will reflect the affective state, being low with depression and normal or high with manic periods.

7. Cerebral thrombosis reveals a decreased blood flow to the region. Following successful bypass surgery blood flow may return to normal.

8. Depending on the variety of brain tumor, changes in oxygen utilization, blood flow, glucose utilization, protein synthesis, and amino acid turnover may be detected. These findings may be helpful in selecting treatment modalities.

9. Obsessive-compulsive disorders may be accompanied by a decreased glucose utilization in the left orbital gyrus of the frontal lobe.

10. Panic episodes, especially in patients who have lactic acid-induced panic, manifest abnor-

mal parahippocampal blood flow, blood volume and oxygen utilization on PET scan. Whole brain metabolism is increased during the panic attack. The hippocampal changes may be related to noradrenergic discharges from the locus ceruleus to the hippocampal area.

Imaging the Neuroleptics on PET

The neuroleptics have a greater affinity for the DA receptor than for other receptors. Therefore, a radio-labeled neuroleptic like chlorpromazine could reveal:

1. The site of the dopaminergic receptors.

2. The density of receptors per unit volume.

3. The affinity of the binding site for the labeled pharmaceutical.

4. The concentration of endogenous agonists available.

Direct interpretation of the image is complicated by certain factors:

1. Neuroleptics bind to other types of receptors.

2. Dopamine receptors themselves have varying affinities for the chlorpromazine molecule.

3. The metabolites of chlorpromazine that retain the positron-emitting isotope might interfere with the image.

4. Since neuroleptics are lipid soluble, there would be nonspecific binding to myelin and other lipids.

Single Photon Tomography

Single photon tomography utilizes radio-labeled I^{23} amphetamine for measuring cerebral blood flow. A rotating gamma camera picks up the photon signal. Tomographic slices of the brain can be constructed in axial, sagittal, coronal, or oblique projections. Unmedicated unipolar depressives have demonstrated a decreased blood flow, while patients with manic disease had an elevated blood flow. The advantage of single photon scanners over PET scanners is that longer-lived isotopes can be employed, making it possible to study larger cortical areas for longer periods of time.

Substance abuse research with the new imaging techniques has been scanty because these studies are only just getting under way. It is predictable that important findings will become available.

Regional Cerebral Blood Flow (rCBF)

Regional CBF measurement relies upon the inhalation or intravenous use of xenon-133, a gamma emitter, in a two-dimensional field. What is actually measured is mean transit time (MTT) after the tracer has been introduced into the bloodstream. Its quantity is measured over a unit of time. The average time that it takes the tracer to traverse the region to be examined is the MTT. Measurement is done by scintillation detectors aimed at the specific region through the skull. Up to 16 detectors are available for each hemisphere. Haloperidol, lithium, or amitriptyline may interfere with accurate readings.

Just how rCBF varies according to local needs is not known at present. Changes in pH may produce regional vasodilation.

The advantages and disadvantages of rCBF are mentioned on the following page.

Advantages	Disadvantages
1. Noninvasive	1. Cortical surface measured only, no deep structures
2. Rapid	
3. Multiple studies are possible because of little radiation exposure	2. Diffuse areas, 2-4 cm, compared to 1 cm by PET

rCBF and Schizophrenia

The question of "hypofrontality" in schizoprenics remains open. It may turn out to be more precisely a matter of dorsolateral prefrontal hypoactivity as seen in rCBF. One report suggests that in unmedicated schizophrenics an increased left hemispheric activation exists when compared to matched controls. This hemispheric difference is corrected by neuroleptic medication which increases right hemisphere blood flow.

The prefrontal cortex, and specifically the dorsolateral segment which is concerned with abstract thinking and decision making, has been studied in chronic schizophrenics and controls. Xenon-133 inhalations were given to determine regional cerebral blood flow. At rest there was no difference in rCBF between the experimental and control groups. When performing a test that specifically required prefrontal lobe functioning, the schizophrenics had no increase in CBF to the area under study while the controls showed a significant increase. The study confirms earlier observations that the prefrontal lobe has a causative role to play in certain schizophrenics. This finding is consistent with the observation that neuroleptic drugs have antipsychotic effects based upon their ability to block nucleus accumbens and other mesolimbic dopaminergic activity. When prefrontal dopamine neurons are lesioned, dopaminergic hypoactivity occurs. Mesolimbic dopaminergic hyperactivity results from loss of inhibition of prefrontal dopaminergic control. Therefore, many instances of schizophrenia can be conceptualized as a hypoactive prefrontal dopamine system which releases dopamine overactivity in the nucleus accumbens. The dorsolateral prefrontal cortex is an area where loss of drive, amotivation, poverty of thought and similar negative symptoms could originate. Therefore, schizophrenics with such symptoms would obtain little relief from neuroleptics since they tend to act on mesolimbic and striatal areas.

Nuclear Magnetic Resonance (NMR); also Magnetic Resonance Imaging (MRI)

The spin orientation of the nuclei of the body's atoms is generally random. When acted upon by a magnetic core they line up in a north-south polar orientation. A radio wave signal at a frequency that will be absorbed by the nucleus of a hydrogen atom is beamed at the tissue, a segment of brain, for example. Magnetic resonance imaging depends upon the hydrogen ion density in the water content of the resonance field of the brain, although certain other magnetic nuclei can be identified at specific radio frequencies. What is imaged is the structure and the energy metabolism of the field.

The advantage of NMR imaging over CT is apparent because the former can distinguish between cortical gray and white matter. Disorders of the white matter which is myelinized, like multiple sclerosis and leukoencephalopathy, can be diagnosed, both being demyelinizing diseases. Other advantages include the lack of ionizing radiation and the fact that iodine-labeled contrast injections are unnecessary.

NMR could provide important information in the area of alcohol research because of the well-known effect of ethanol on neuronal membranes. With NMR the capability of examining alcohol-induced membrane perturbations and the partitioning of alcohol between the membrane and the cytoplasm is possible. One study of patients with Wernicke's disease was able to diagnose atrophy of the mamillary bodies, a finding frequently made at autopsy. Cerebral edema and infarction have been diagnosed with the NMR imaging technique.

NMR and Schizophrenia

Every imaging technique has provided some support for the hypofrontality hypothesis of schizophrenia, although negative investigations are also available. A recent NMR study of young schizophrenic men and age-matched controls revealed markedly smaller frontal lobes in 40% of the schizophrenic group. The decrease was found in the dorsolateral and orbital regions of the frontal lobe. No relationship was found between frontal lobe size and negative symptoms or the ability to perform frontal lobe function tests. In addition, a decreased cranial and cerebral size was noted on sagittal NMR scans, indicating the possibility of some genetic or early environmental developmental dysplasia.

Brain Electrical Activity Mapping (BEAM)

The BEAM technique provides color maps of computed electrical activity of the brain. The images are derived from 25 gold electrodes applied to the scalp, which are amplified through a 20-channel polygraph and recorded on a 28-channel FM analog tape recorder. Artifacts are eliminated. Spectral analysis is performed. Each electrode production is analyzed for alpha, beta, delta, and theta activity. The brain is fairly completely mapped for electrical activity.

Evoked potentials are generated to random light flashes. Each electrode site is measured for the evoked potential voltage, which can be topographically mapped in color.

Both medicated and unmedicated schizophrenic patients had increased bilateral electroencephalographic delta activity somewhat more marked over frontal areas as compared to controls. The bilateral slowing of the spectral analyzed EEG especially in the frontal lobes in schizophrenics has been confirmed in a number of studies, but not in all.

Many other uses of the BEAM are possible. In fact, it actually represents an important refinement of the EEG.

Magnetoencephalography (MEG)

The electrical and magnetic fields generated by the brain are the product of nerve cell action, essentially of their membrane potentials. When a discrete population of neurons is activated, the magnetic field which is produced remains localized to the region of its origin. The magnetic field of a neuron or an assembly of neurons is very weak. A highly sensitive magnetic sensor is required, and one that must reject background "noise." The MEG is able to show the sites of electrical activity as a function of time. It can identify one or more magnetic brain signals in three dimensions within a few millimeters. Up to 100 channels are capable of development.

The primary use of MEG is for the localization of focal epilepsy. During the period between seizures, isolated electrical spikes can be seen on the MEG. They are of importance because the exact location of an epileptic focus for surgical excision can be derived by MEG. Since the movement of an electromagnetic neuronal impulse can be followed by MEG, other potential applications of this technique in addition to epilepsy are being explored.

7

Future Prospects

During the coming years neurochemists, neurophysiologists, neuropharmacologists, and other scientists will continue their search into the nature of the brain. It is predictable that many significant discoveries will be uncovered. Considering the current preoccupation with brain function and the available advanced technologies, new knowledge will come forth at an accelerated rate.

What will we learn? We will learn that understanding the mind is more complicated than we even now imagine. Although simplifying general principles will become discernible, the sheer complexity of mental function at every level will become evident.

It should not be assumed that the massive convolutions of the chemical activities within the CNS are sufficiently revealed in this volume. Only the major effects of drugs have been presented here; lesser effects have not been described. The multiplicity of neurotransmitter interactions on involved human processes such as memory, learning, sexuality, feeding or sleeping are abundant indeed. This marvel of complexity, even at our present level of ignorance, is impressive.

As we come to understand the substrate of cognitive and emotional disorders, it will follow that superior neuroleptics, anxiolytics, antidepressants, and antiphobics will be developed. Whether character disorders are to become manageable by psychochemicals is less evident.

As an example of how improved drug therapies can improve the treatment situation, neuroleptics that provide a discrete dopaminergic blockade of the limbic system would be an important advance. If a dopaminergic effect on the striatal area could be avoided, chemical Parkinsonism and tardive dyskinesia would not be a problem. Side effects like blurred vision, dry mouth, urinary retention and sedation are caused by antimuscarinic activity of the neuroleptics. The antimuscarinic action is not needed for the antipsychotic properties of these agents. Nor do the alpha adrenergic effects contribute to the primary purpose of neuroleptics. They only lead to adverse reactions such as postural hypotension, dizziness, and sedation. If such untoward complications of the neuroleptics could be eliminated, higher doses for patients who might need them will become more feasible. Patient compliance would improve if the adverse side effects which now lead to abandonment of therapy were no longer present. Drugs of the future designed for very precise actions in circumscribed brain areas are by no means impossible. In fact, such developments might be expected.

Entirely new drug classes may come forth as a result of continuing research efforts. Antieuphoriants, for example, may be helpful in selected cases of cocaine dependence to eliminate the rewarding aspects of that drug. Naltrexone is, in effect, an antieuphoriant for heroin, and it is useful for some patients. The neuroleptics will block much of the cocaine euphoria, but the problem is one of compliance. If a neuroleptic with a low level of undesirable side effects were available, it could contribute to efforts to deal with cocaine dependency problems.

Considering the extension of the life span in this century, a great need exists for an antidementing agent. Before such a medication could be effective, a method of achieving a much earlier diagnosis of the dementias will be necessary. At present the diagnosis is usually made long after substantial structural changes have occurred. The PET scan or its successor may permit identification of the dementing disorders before symptoms appear above the clinical horizon.

A more somber side to the study of the chemical brain is

a concern for the future, but it is already here in a precursory form. Until recently, certain botanicals were the traditional sources of awareness-altering drugs. Manufactured substances such as amphetamines and barbiturates were added in this century as abused items. However, these chemicals arrived on the street through medical channels so that scrutiny of their toxicity was fairly well established.

Now, and inevitably in the future, we will be confronted with a situation in which analogues of currently used and abused drugs will displace the customary mind-altering potions. Some of them are of unusual potency and all are completely untested insofar as their toxic potential is concerned.

Some of these "designer drugs" are not scheduled under the Controlled Substances Act. Others have been hastily scheduled, but with the result that a new, unscheduled analogue came forth. The number of minor manipulations of the basic molecular structure that can be produced is great.

One such agent, MPPP, manufactured specifically for the illicit trade, has caused permanent disability and death. Because of a minor error in its synthesis, a related chemical, MPTP, was created, which caused death of dopaminergic neurons and inevitable, fulminating Parkinsonism. Another opioid, 3-methylfentanyl, has produced a number of overdose deaths because it was so difficult to properly measure the dosage. This is a thousand times more potent than heroin. Still another "designer drug" has the possibility of long-term toxicity, namely loss of serotonin-producing cells. That drug is Ecstasy, MDMA.

These drugs are offered on the black market without quality controls, safety testing, or fiscal responsibility for any damage that may be incurred. Users permit chemical intrusions into their central nervous system by chemists who have no particular concern for them. Pollution of this sort, of the internal environment, is an offense against consumers far worse than any pollution of the external environment.

The ability of our street chemists to improve on nature is unquestioned. What is fascinating is that millions of people, otherwise concerned about their well-being, allow themselves to become human guinea pigs for whatever product the garage psychochemist proffers.

The exploration of the chemical brain will surely continue. We are much closer to the beginning than to the end of this search. The molecular diseases of the mind will predictably be resolved by genetic engineering, brain imaging, immunohistochemical mapping, gene cloning and by drugs that mimic the naturally occurring neuropeptides. Disorders of memory, learning and behavior are being approached on many neurobiological fronts with some expectation that emerging techniques will improve many of these defective conditions. This is an exciting time to be a student of the mind.

And, as we press on, we must continue to ask one question—a question whose answer cannot and will not be provided by science alone, but rather by all of us, as we constitute an informed and compassionate society: Why, if the brain-mind is so unique and its fullest potential not yet explored, do we clumsily attempt to manipulate it with alcohol and dubious chemicals?

Glossary

ACh - Acetylcholine, a neurotransmitter.

adenylate cyclase - An enzyme that catalyzes the conversion of ATP to cAMP.

agonist - A chemical that acts like a neurotransmitter.

agonist-antagonist - A chemical that has both agonistic and antagonistic effects. Usually, it has agonistic actions on one subtype of receptor and antagonistic effects on another subtype of receptor.

alpha waves - EEG waves with a frequency of 8-13/sec., indicating a resting state.

anhedonia - The inability to feel pleasure.

antagonist - A chemical that has an effect opposite to a neurotransmitter.

antigen - A substance capable of inducing a specific immune response.

astrocytes - Glial cells that support neurons and form the blood-brain barrier, barring certain molecules access to the brain.

ATP - Adenosine triphosphate, a nucleotide which has high energy phosphate bonds to provide energy for cell metabolism, a second messenger.

autoreceptors - Receptors on the presynaptic neuron that provide feedback information from the postsynaptic cell.

axon - Axons transmit impulses from the cell body to other nerve cells. They are single but may branch and are usually covered by a myelin sheath provided by glial cells.

axon terminal - Also bouton or synaptic terminal. At the distal end of the axon, a knoblike bulge that contains many transmitter vesicles.

BEAM - Brain electrical activity mapping, an imaging device.

beta waves - EEG waves with a frequency of 18-30/sec., present during the alert state.

bipolar affective disorder - Manic-depressive psychosis, characterized by major mood swings.

bouton - The enlarged end of the axon.

C_3 wave - A negative defection of the ERP C_3 wave, perhaps a marker for inherited alcoholism.

Ca^{++} - Calcium ion.

cAMP - Cyclic adenosine monophosphate, a nucleotide second messenger, formed from ATP by the action of adenylate cyclase.

catecholamines - Those transmitter amines related to catechol, namely, dopamine, norepinephrine and epinephrine.

CCK - Cholecystokinin, an intestinal hormone and neurohormone.

cell body - Also soma and perikaryon. The enlarged area of a neuron which contains the nucleus and cytoplasmic contents which manufacture essential cellular contents.

cGMP - Cyclic guanosine monophosphate, a second messenger.

Cl^- - Chloride ion.

CNS - The central nervous system which includes the brain and spinal cord. The autonomic nervous system (ANS) innervates the viscera, and the peripheral nervous system consists of the nerves that go to the skin, muscles, and bones.

COMT - Catechol-O-methyltransferase, a metabolizing enzyme.

corpus striatum - A part of the extrapyramidal system containing the caudate nucleus, the putamen and the globus pallidus.

CT - Computed tomography, also CAT, computerized axial tomography, an imaging device.

DA - Dopamine, a neurotransmitter.

DAT - Dementia of the Alzheimer type.

delta waves - EEG waves with a frequency of less than 4/sec. Slow waves typical of deep sleep.

dendrite - Dendrites are single or multiple fibers extending from the cell body that branch into treelike structures. They receive chemical information from the axons of other neurons.

demyelinization - The loss of the myelin sheath formed by glial cells around the axon. The loss of myelin causes slowed and aberrant neural transmission.

deoxyglucose - A glucose analogue which is longer lasting in the brain than glucose. It is therefore labeled and used for PET scans when glucose utilization studies will extend beyond the time available if glucose were used.

depolarized - Discharged, ion current generated.

detoxification - The removal of a dependency-producing drug from a person who has become tolerant to it. Depressant drugs usually require gradual discontinuance. Stimulant drugs can be stopped abruptly.

DNA - Deoxyribonucleic acid, a nucleotide, exists in all cells and carries genetic information in all organisms except the RNA viruses.

dopa - Dihydroxyphenylalanine, a precursor to DA.

downregulation - A decrease in receptor sites caused when excessive numbers of transmitter molecules are available to the receptor over time.

dysphoria - Displeasure, unhappiness, and similar noxious feelings.

dysplasia - Abnormal structural development.

E - Epinephrine, adrenaline, a neurotransmitter.

endogenous opioid peptides - The internally derived opioids from amino acid linkages that form three types of peptides: enkephalins, endorphins and dynorphins. These are, in turn, derived from larger peptides: proenkephalins, proopiomelanocortins and prodynorphins.

endoplasmic reticulum - The area in the cell body that manufactures peptides, proteins and neurotransmitters, also known as the smooth endoplasmic reticulum.

endorphin - Particularly beta endorphin, a potent internally produced peptide analgesic many times more potent than morphine. In this book "endorphin" is also used generically to designate all endogenous opioids.

endothelium - The inner layer of cells that lines the blood vessels.

epinephrine - (also adrenaline) - A peripheral and central nervous system transmitter.

ERP - Event-related potential, electrical recording from a single sensory stimulus. Also EP.

euphorohallucinogens - Drugs which stand between mescaline and amphetamine in chemical structure. In small doses they tend to be euphoriants, and in large amounts hallucinogenic effects become evident.

extrapyramidal syndrome (EPS) - The movement disorder that is associated with aging, the use of neuroleptics, MPTP, carbon monoxide, etc. It consists of cogwheel rigidity, tremors, weakness, drooling, expressionless face, loss of associated movements, stooped posture, and a festinating gait. Also Parkinsonism and paralysis agitans (obs.).

extrapyramidal system (EPS) - A functional system of motor neurons, excluding the direct motor system of the pyramidal tracts. It controls posture, gait, and fine movements. It includes the corpus striatum, the substantia nigra, the red nucleus and their extensions.

false transmitter - A substance, often an amine, that can be stored in presynaptic vesicles and released or occupies but has little or no effect on the postsynaptic receptors.

5-HIAA - 5-hydroxyindolacetic acid, end product of 5-HT metabolism.

5-HT - 5-hydroxytryptamine, serotonin, a neurotransmitter.

focal epilepsy - Minor seizures that present with myoclonic jerks without loss of consciousness.

FSH - Follicle-stimulating hormone, synthesized in the anterior pituitary, stimulates growth and maturation of the ovum.

GABA - Gamma aminobutyric acid, an inhibitory neurotransmitter.

GAD - Glutamic acid decarboxylase, a GABA enzyme.

galactorrhea - The secretion of milk in a nonpregnant individual.

glia - Cells that support and provide nourishment to neurons in the CNS.

GnRH - Gonadotropin-releasing hormone.

Golgi apparatus - Packages of transmitters, peptides and proteins made by the endoplasmic reticulum placed within vesicles to prevent their metabolism. Also called rough endoplasmic reticulum.

H - Histamine, a monoamine transmitter.

hippocampus (literally, sea horse) - A curved elevation at the floor of the lateral ventricle involved with memory and learning processes.

Huntington's disease - A hereditary disease characterized by a progressive chorea and dementia.

HVA - Homovanillic acid, an end product of dopamine metabolism.

hyperpolarized - Unable to discharge, excessive negativity.

hypofrontality - A diminished structure and function of the prefrontal cortex sometimes associated with schizophrenia.

hypothalamus - A brain region near the pituitary gland that regulates water balance, body temperature, sleep, food intake and the development of secondary sexual characteristics. Secretes hormone releasing and inhibiting factors controlling the pituitary.

ictal - An epileptic episode.

ion - The dissociation of a chemical into atoms or radicals that have a positive (anion) or negative (cation) charge.

ion channels - Pores in neuron membranes specific for each ion.

K^{++} - Potassium ion.

Korsakoff's encephalopathy - See Wernicke's encephalopathy.

L-dopa - (levo-dihydroxyphenylalanine, also levodopa) A precursor of DA, NE and E.

leukoencephalopathy - A disorder caused by a defect in the formation and maintenance of the myelin sheath.

LH - Luteinizing hormone, synthesized in the anterior pituitary, causes ovulation and the secretion of estrogen.

ligand - A molecule that acts in the same manner as a neurotransmitter.

limbic system - Consisting of the amygdala, the hippocampus, the hypothalamus, the septum, the cingulate gyrus and their extensions. the system is involved in emotion and its integration with cognition.

lipid - Fats and related compounds that are insoluble in water and soluble in volatile solvents.

locus ceruleus - A blue spot in the pons, the site of most NE cell bodies with connections throughout the brain.

LSD - Lysergic acid diethylamide, a hallucinogen.

maintenance - Maintaining a fairly consistent dose of an opioid over a period of months or years as a means of keeping the patient in treatment and off illicit opioids.

MAO - Monoamine oxidase, a monoamine enzyme.

MDA - Methylene dioxyamphetamine, also the Love Drug, a euphorohallucinogen.

MDMA - Methylene dioxymethamphetamine, also Ecstacy, a euphorhallucinogen.

MEG - Magnetoencephalography, an imaging device.

MHPG - 3-methoxy-4-hydroxyphenylglycol, an end product of NE metabolism.

microtubules - Minute tubules along the axon which permit delivery of a variety of substances protected from enzyme breakdown. Also used for retrograde molecular flow.

miosis - Constricted pupils.

mitochondria - Intracellular structures that provide energy by means of high energy bonds like ATP.

monoamines - The transmitter amines that have single amine groups: DA, NE, E, H and 5-HT.

MPPP - 1-methyl-4-phenyl-4-propionoxypiperdine, related to meperidine, a synthetic opioid. Sold on the street as synthetic heroin.

MPTP - 1-methyl-4-phenyl-1,2,3,6-tetrahydropyridine, a toxic compound produced in an erroneous synthesis of MPPP. Causes severe Parkinsonism.

mRNA - A template of DNA that conveys information from DNA to protein-forming systems in the cell, also messenger RNA.

myelin - The lipid cell membrane of the oligodendrocyte that forms a myelin sheath around the axon, increasing the signal speed.

Na$^+$ - Sodium ion.

NE - Norepinephrine, a neurotransmitter.

neurohormone - A neurohormone acts on distant receptor target cells following its release into the extracellular fluid or bloodstream. A neurohormone may act as a neurotransmitter at one synapse but can have modulator or hormonal effects at other sites that possess its receptors.

neuroleptic - Also antipsychotic and major tranquilizer. A compound that reduces the symptoms of psychosis, particularly schizophrenia. It usually is a dopamine receptor blocker.

neuromodulator - Neuromodulators act at a local or distant postsynaptic site to modify a neurotransmitter's activity or rate of release, amplifying or attenuating its effect.

NMI - Nuclear magnetic imaging, also NMR.

NMR - Nuclear magnetic resonance, an imaging device.

nucleus accumbens - A dopaminergic projection system, a reward center, and perhaps related to schizophrenia.

oligodendrocytes - Glial cells that form the myelin sheaths (white matter) that surround the axon.

opiates - An obsolescent term that delineated opium and derivatives of opium.

opioids - All members of a class of compounds that act similarly to morphine that is; they produce analgesia, sedation, and drive reduction. This includes derivatives of opium, synthetic drugs, and endogenous peptides that occupy opiopeptide binding sites.

opiopeptide - An enkephalin, endorphin or dynorphin peptide.

PCP - Phenylcyclohexylpiperdine, also phencyclidine and Sernyl, a synthetic, hallucinogenic-anesthetic drug.

peptide - A molecule containing two or more amino acids with an amine group at one end of the peptide chain and a carboxyl group at the other.

PET - Positron emission tomography, an imaging device.

pH - The relative acidity of a biologic fluid, with acidic solutions having a pH below 7 and alkaline solutions having a pH above 7.

pineal body - A small, cone-shaped gland lying below the corpus callosum, a site of melatonin synthesis. Control over biological rhythmic activities originates here.

pinocytosis - Tiny invaginations of the cell membrane which take up molecules of a transmitter substance from the synapses, then close to form vesicles.

polarized - Able to discharge, has an action potential.

postsynaptic membrane - The membrane, usually on a dendrite, that receives the neurotransmitter at its receptor site.

potentiator - A drug which when used with another drug produces an effect greater than the sum of each drug used alone.

presynaptic membrane - The membrane of an axon terminal which delivers transmitters into the synapse by exocytosis, and later retrieves free transmitters by a molecular pump.

raphe - A series of 5-HT nuclei that extends from the midline of the medulla to the pons. It sends fibers to the pineal gland, the hypothalamus, the cerebellum and the cerebral cortex.

rCBF - Regional cerebral blood flow.

receptor site - Also affinity, binding, or recognition site. The stereospecific acceptor lipoprotein for the transmitter delivered across the synapse.

reinforcement - Increasing the response to a stimulus by providing a reward, alternatively decreasing the response by providing punishment.

REM - Rapid eye movement sleep, dreaming sleep.

second messenger - A substance that transmits cellular information following arrival of the initial message at the postsynaptic receptor site.

serotonin - 5-hydroxytryptamine, a neurotransmitter.

single photon tomography - A special form of PET scan.

striatum - Also corpus striatum. A component of the basal ganglia lying in front of the thalamus. Functionally it is part of the EPS, controlling muscle tone.

substantia nigra - A small black area in the midbrain which is the origin of many dopaminergic neurons.

sympathomimetic - Derived from the autonomic sympathetic nervous system, also adrenergic.

synapse - Also synaptic cleft. A space between neurons about 20 nanometers (20 billionths of a meter) wide through which neurotransmitters pass to transmit chemical information. The usual synapse is axodendritic (axon to dendrite) although other types occur.

tardive dyskinesia - A movement disorder marked by involuntary, repetitive movements of the tongue, mouth and face induced by long-term use of neuroleptics, which produce dopamine blockade, then sensitization of dopamine receptors.

TCA - Tricyclic antidepressants, the major group of drugs used in the treatment of depression.

terminal bouton - Also axon terminal. A bulge of the axon in the vicinity of the synapse. It contains the synaptic vesicles which enclose the neurotransmitter.

THC - Tetrahydrocannabinol, the active ingredient in marijuana.

theta waves - EEG waves with a frequency of 4-7/sec. Slow waves typical of sleep or drowsiness.

tyrosine hydroxylase - An enzyme that converts tyrosine to dopa. The rate-limiting step in the synthesis of catecholamines.

unipolar depression - Depression which does not cycle with manic episodes. May be a part of a bipolar disorder, but mania has not yet become manifest.

upregulation - An increase in receptor sites caused when decreased numbers of transmitter molecules are available.

ventral tegmentum - An area near the substantia nigra in the midbrain and pons containing dopaminergic cell bodies with extensions to reward areas and the EPS.

vesicle - A tiny sac containing molecules of transmitter substances in the presynaptic terminal.

Wernicke's disease (also Wernicke-Korsakoff disease) - A thiamine deficiency disorder most often seen in chronic alcoholics and manifested by dementia, eye muscle paralysis, polyneuritis, and severe loss of recent memory.

Additional Readings

The Chemical Neuron

Bloom, F.E., Lazerson, A. and Hofstadler, L. *Brain, Mind and Behavior*. W.H. Freeman Co., New York, 1985.

Cooper, J.R., Bloom, F.E. and Roth, R.H. *The Biochemical Basis of Neuropharmacology*. Oxford University Press, Oxford, 1986.

Goldstein, G.W. and Betz, A.L. The Blood-Brain Barrier. *Scientific American*. 235: 74-83, 1986.

Marx, J.L. Nerve growth factor acts in brain. *Science*. 232: 1341-1342, 1986.

The Neuroscience of Mental Health. NIMH. American Psychiatric Press. Washington, D.C., undated.

Thompson, R.F. *The Brain*. W.H. Freeman Co., New York, 1985.

Neurotransmitters, Neuropeptides and Neurohormones

P.H. Abelson, *Neuroscience*. E. Butz, and S.H. Snyder (Eds.). A.A.A.S., Washington, D.C., 1985.

Baskin, Y. The way we act. *Science*. 85: 94-101, 1985.

Baulsfield, G. *Neurotransmitters in Action*. Elsevir, New York, 1984.

Bradford, H.F. *Chemical Neurobiology*. W. H. Freeman Co., New York, 1986.

Coyle, J.T. (Ed.). *An Introduction to the World of Neurotransmitters and Neuroreceptors*. In: APA Annual Reviews, Vol. H, R.E. Hales and A.J. Frances (Eds.), 1985.

D'Amato, R.J. et al. Selectivity of the Parkinsonian neurotoxin, MPTP: toxic metabolite MPP+ binds to neuromelanin. *Science*. 231: 987-989, 1986.

Ferreto, P. et al. *Neuropharmacology*. 23: 1359, 1984.

Gilman, A.G. and Goodman, L.S. (Eds.). *The Pharmacological Basis of Therapeutics, VII Edition*. Macmillan, New York, 1985.

Lipton, M.A., DiMascio, A., and Killam, K. *Psychophar-macology: A Generation of Progress*. Raven Press, New York, 1978.

Meyer, F.B. Selective central nervous system blockers — a new class of anticonvulsant agents. *Mayo Clinic Proceedings*. 61: 239-247, 1986.

Pankepp, J. The neurochemistry of behavior. In: *Annual Review of Psychology, Vol. 37*. M.R. Rosenzweig and W.P. Lyman (Eds.) Annual Reviews, 4139 El Camino Way, Palo Alto, CA, 1986.

Pfeiffer, A. et al. Psychotomimesis mediated by K opiate receptor. *Science*. 233: 774-776, 1986.

Squire, L.R. Mechanisms of memory. *Science*. 232: 1612-1618, 1986.

Stahl, S.M. et al. Neurochemistry of dopamine in Huntington's dementia and normal aging. *Science*. 43: 161-164, 1986.

Zucker, R.S. and Lands, L. Mechanism of transmitter release: Voltage hypothesis and calcium hypothesis. *Science*. 231: 514-579, 1986.

The Chemistry of Addiction

Cocaine Use in American: Epidemiologic and Clinical Perspectives. N.J. Kozel and E.H. Adams (Eds.), NIDA Research Monograph #61, U.S. Gov't. Printing Office, Washington, D.C. 20402, 1985.

Costa, H.A.E. Diazepam-binding inhibitor: A neuropeptide located in selected neuronal populations of rat brain. *Science*. 229: 179-182, 1985.

Drug Abuse and Drug Abuse Research. First Triennial Report to the Congress. HHS, NIDA, Rockville, MD., Publ. No. (ADMC) 85-1372, 1984.

Drug Abuse and Drug Abuse Research. Second Triennial Report to the Congress. HHS, NIDA, Rockville, MD, to be published, 1987.

Freedman, D.X. Hallucinogenic drug research: If so, so what? *Pharmacology, Biochemistry & Behavior*. 24: 407-415, 1986.

Gawin, F.H. and Kleber, H.D. Abstinence symptomatology and psychiatric diagnosis in cocaine abusers. *Arch. Gen. Psychiatry.* 43: 107-113, 1986.

Goldstein, A. Brain chemistry and the addictions. Presented at the Sidney Cohen Lectureship, Los Angeles, CA, 1986.

Goodwin, D.W. Alcoholism and heredity. *Arch. Gen. Psychiatry.* 36: 57-61, 1979.

Martin, B.M. Pharmacokinetics and mechanism of action of phencyclidine. Symposium presented by the American Society for Pharmacology and Experimental Therapeutics, New Orleans, 1982.

Martin, P.R. et al. Response to ethanol reduced by past thiamine deficiency. *Science.* 227: 1385-1388, 1985.

Millman, R.E. (Ed.). *Drug Abuse and Drug Dependence.* In: APA Annual Review, Vol. 5, R.E. Hales and A.J. Frances, (Eds.), American Psychiatric Press, Washington, D.C., 1985.

Neuroscience Methods in Drug Abuse Research. R.M. Brown, D.P. Friedman and Y. Nimit (Eds.) NIDA Research Monograph #62, U.S. Gov't. Printing Office, Washington, D.C. 20402, 1985.

Problems of Drug Dependence, 1985. L.S. Harris, (Ed.) Research Monograph #67, U.S. Gov't. Printing Office, Washington, D.C. 20402, 1986.

Snyder, S.N. Drug and neurotransmitter receptors in the brain. *Science.* 224: 22-34, 1984.

Szara, S. *Neurobiology of Behavioral Control in Drug Abuse.* NIDA Research Monograph #74, U.S. Gov't. Printing Office, Washington, D.C. 20402, 1986.

The Pharmacotherapy of Addictions

Blum, K. *Handbook of Abusable Drugs.* Gardener Press, New York, 1984.

Cocaine: Pharmacology, Effects and Treatment of Abuse., J. Grabowski (Ed.), NIDA Research Monograph #50, U.S. Gov't. Printing Office, Washington, D.C. 20402, 1984.

Cohen, S. *The Substance Abuse Problems, Vol. II*. Hayworth Press, New York, 1985.

Dackis, C.A. and Gold, M. Pharmacologic approaches to cocaine addiction. *J. Substance Abuse Treatment*. 2: 139-147, 1985.

Kleber, H.D. Naltrexone. *J. Substance Abuse Treatment*. 2: 117-122, 1985.

LAAM: Technical Review. National Institute on Drug Abuse, Rockville, MD, 1983.

Lowinson, J.H. and Ruiz, P. (Eds.). *Substance Abuse: Clinical Problems and Perspectives*. Williams & Wilkins, Baltimore, 1981.

Phencyclidine: An Update. D.H. Clouet (Ed.), NIDA Research, Monograph #64, NIDA, 5600 Fishers Lane, Rockville, MD 20857, 1986.

Snyder, S.H. *Drugs and the Brain*. W.H. Freeman Co., Salt Lake City, 1986.

The Genetics of Substance Abuse

Alcoholism: An Inherited Disease. DHHS Publ. No. ADM85-1426. U.S. Gov't. Printing Office, Washington, D.C. 20402, 1985.

Ebihara, S. et al. Genetic control of melatonin synthesis in the pineal gland of the mouse. *Science*. 231: 491-493, 1985.

Genetic and Biological Markers in Drug Abuse and Alcoholism. M.C. Braude and H.M. Chao. (Eds.), NIDA Research Monograph #66. U.S. Gov't. Printing Office, Washington, D.C. 20402, 1986.

Goodwin, D.W. The genetics of alcoholism. *Substance and Alcohol Misuse/Abuse*. 1: 101-117, 1980.

Goodwin, D.W. Alcoholism and genetics. *Arch. Gen. Psychiatry*. 42: 171-174, 1985.

Imaging the Brain

Andreasen, N. et al. Structural abnormalities in the frontal system in schizophrenia. *Arch. Gen. Psychiatry*. 43: 136-144, 1986.

Barth, D.S. et al. Neuromagnetic localization of epileptiform spike activity in human brain. *Science*. 891-894, 1982.

Barth, D.S. et al. Neuromagnetic evidence of spatially disturbed sources underlying epileptiform spikes in the human brain. *Science*. 223: 293-296, 1984.

Beatty, J. et al. Magnetically localizing the sources of epileptic discharges within the human brain. *Naval Research Reviews*. 36: 20-28, 1984.

Beresford, T.P. CT scanning in psychiatric inpatients: Clinical yield. *Psychosomatics*. 27: 105-112, 1986.

Berman, K.F. et al. Physiologic dysfunction of dorsolateral prefrontal cortex in schizophrenia. *Arch. Gen. Psychiatry*. 43: 126-134, 1986.

Bibliography on Imaging Technology. L.L. Faudin and H.M. Chao (Eds.) Rockville, MD, 1986.

DeLisi, L.E. et al. A family study of the association of increased ventricular size with schizophrenia. *Arch. Gen. Psychiatry*. 43: 148-153, 1986.

Frytak, S. et al. Magnetic resonance imaging for neurotoxicity in long term survivors of carcinoma. *Mayo Clinic Proceedings*. 60: 803-879, 1986.

Goetz, K.L. and van Kammen, D.P. Computerized axial tomography scans and subtypes of schizophrenia. *J. Nerv. Mental Dis*. 174: 31-41, 1986.

Morihisa, J.M. *Brain Imagining in Psychiatry*. American Psychiatric Press, Washington, D.C., 1984.

Nasrallah, H.A., et al. Cerebral ventricular enlargement in schizophrenia. *Arch. Gen. Psychiatry*. 43: 157-159, 1986.

Phelps, M.E. and Mazziotta, J.C. Positron emission tomography: Human brain function and biochemistry. *Science*. 228: 799-809, 1985.

Weinberger, D.R. et al. Physiologic dysfunction of dorsolateral prefrontal cortex in schizophrenia. *Arch. Gen. Psychiatry*. 43: 114-124, 1986.